FOOD FACTS, MYTHS
AND HEALTHY DIETS

Other books related to nutrition by
Professor Devareddy Narahari include:

Cholesterol Myths and Facts

Cholesterol, Fats and Healthy Diets

Agro-forestry Products (Herbs) in Foods and Feeds

Chicken Fast Foods—Preservation and Quality Control

FOOD FACTS, MYTHS AND HEALTHY DIETS

Prof. Devareddy Narahari, Ph.D

Book design and book cover by Jean Boles
jean.bolesbooks@gmail.com
https://www.upwork.com/fl/jeanboles

Dedication

*This book is dedicated to **our mother Earth** and to **my parents**, who brought me into this world; to all my **teachers**, who taught me this science; and to my **relatives, friends and well-wishers**, who inspired me to write this book. I humbly submit this book to **GOD**.*

Contents

List of Abbreviations Used in the Text

ACSH: American Council on Science and Health

ADA: American Dietetic Association

AHA: s Association

AJCN: American Journal of Clinical Nutrition

ALA: Alpha Linoleic Acid (C18:3/ α n-3 /Ω 3- fatty acid)

BMI: Body Mass Index

BMR/RMR: Basal Metabolic Rate / Resting Metabolic Rate

BNF: British Nutrition Foundation

CDCS: Center for Disease Control and Prevention

CFTRI: Central Food Technology Research Institute (Mysore, India)

CHD: Coronary Heart Disease

CHO: Carbohydrates (starch & sugars)

CMAFN: Committee on Medical Aspects of Food and Nutrition

CNS: Chinese Nutrition Society

COMA: Committee on Medical Aspects of Food Policy

CVD: Cardio Vascular Diseases

DHA: Dicosa Hexa-Enoic Acid (C22:6, a n-3 /Ω 3- fatty acid)

DPA: Dicosa Penta-Enoic Acid (C22:5, a n-3 /Ω 3- fatty acid)

DHSS: Department of Health and Social Security of UK

EAA: Essential Amino Acids

EFA: Essential Fatty Acids

EFSA: European Food Society Authority

ENC: Egg and Nutrition Center

EPA: Eicosa Penta-Enoic Acid (C20:5, a n-3 /Ω 3- fatty acid)

FAO: Food and Agriculture Organization of the United Nations

FFA: Free Fatty Acids

FDA: Federal Drug Administration of USA

FSIS: Food Safety and Inspection Service

HDLC: High Density Lipoprotein (bound) Cholesterol (good cholesterol)

IBS: Irritable Bowel Syndrome

ICMR: Indian Council of Medical Research

ION: Institute of Optimal Nutrition, UK

LDLC:Low Density Lipoprotein (bound) Cholesterol (bad cholesterol)

LPIMIC: Linus Pauling Institute's Micronutrient Information Center of Oregon State University

Lipids: Includes fats, oils, fat soluble vitamins, cholesterol and other fat soluble substances

LRCP: Lipid Research Clinics Programme

MRFIT: Multiple Risk Factor Intervention Trail Research group

MUFA: Mono Unsaturated Fatty Acids (Ω-9 FA- mostly Oleic acid)

NAS: National Academy of Sciences

NCCAAHA: Nutrition Committee & Council on Arteriosclerosis of American Heart Association

NCEP: National Cholesterol Education Programme

NCEPHLBI: National Cholesterol Education Programme of the Heart, Lung & Blood Institute

NCIA: National Cancer Institute of America

NFC: National Fiber Council

NIH: National Institute of Health

NIN: National Institute of Nutrition (Hyderabad, India)

List of Abbreviations Used in the Text

NRC: National Research Council of USA

n-3 /n-6 / n-9 or Ω-3, 6, 9 FA: Omega (Ω)-3 / 6 / 9 fatty acids

NSP: Non-Starch Poly-saccharides (fiber)

PUFA: Poly Unsaturated Fatty Acids (Ω-3 & 6 FA)

RCPL: Royal College of Physicians of London

RDA: Recommended Daily Allowances

SFA: Saturated Fatty Acids

TFA: Trans Fatty Acids

TGL: Triglycerides

USDA: United States Department of Agriculture

USDHHS: United States Department of Health & Human Services

VLDLC: Very Low Density Lipoprotein (bound) Cholesterol

WHO: World Health Organization

Acknowledgements

I am highly grateful to ADA, AHA, BNF, CNS, CMAFN, COMA, EFSA, ENC, FAO, FDA, ICMR, ION, LPIMIC, NAS, NCCAAHA, NCEP, NCIA, NFC, NIH, NIN, NRC, RCPL, USDA, USDHHS, WHO and various universities and research centers for the opportunity of utilizing some of their data, information and findings at appropriate places while writing this book. I sincerely acknowledge the valid lectures and articles of Drs. Barron, Bereliani, Berg, Briffa, Dugoua, Haas, Hyman, Keith, Lundell, Lustig, Mercola, Oz, Radha Iyyar, Wolfson and many more, which inspired me to undertake this work. I am also thankful to some of the commercial organizations, and to my friends and family members for motivating me to write this book on health and nutrition.

Dr. Devareddy Narahari

Preface

In developing countries, the scientific information available and the dietary guidelines suggested by the health authorities are most often the replica of those from developed countries, where the food and food habits are entirely different. Hence, the dietary guidelines and recommendations suggested by them may not be suitable for the population in developing countries. Following those guidelines at many times may lead to negative results and newer health problems. This book is published to provide updated information on food and nutrition to the public, based on the existing environment, foods, food habits and lifestyle.

This book also deals with several nutrition-related myths that may be in the minds of the public and replaces these myths with facts. The information given in this book is not only the author's opinion; it is based on the latest and authenticated statistical, demographical and research information collected from the Food and Agriculture Organization of the United Nations (FAO); United States Department of Agriculture (USDA); Indian Council of Medical Research (ICMR); National Institute of Nutrition (NIN); Multiple Risk Factor Intervention Trail (MRFIT) Research group; Committee on Medical Aspects of Food Policy (COMA); American Heart Association (AHA); American Dietetic Association (ADA); National Research Council (NRC); American Council on Science and Health; Department of Health and Social Security (DHSS) of UK; Lipid Research Clinics Program (LRCP); Nutrition Committee and Council on Arteriosclerosis of the American Heart Association (NCCAAHA); National Cholesterol Education Program of the Heart, Lung and Blood Institute

(NCEPHLBI) of USA; Committee on Medical Aspects of Food and Nutrition (CMAFN) Government of UK; Egg and Nutrition Center (ENC); Federal Drug Administration of USA (FDA); Food Safety and Inspection Service (FSIS); Institute of Optimal Nutrition, UK (ION); and various universities, research centers and other health--nutrition authorities from many countries across the world.

The multiple data collected from different sources were subjected to meta-analysis, meticulously interpreted, with logical and scientific reasoning linked with present day actual food habits and life style, to arrive at valid conclusions. This information will be useful for people all over the world in helping them to select the right kind of balanced food. It will also give sufficient scientific information to the local health and nutrition authorities for recommending correct dietary guidelines and suggesting recommended daily allowances (RDA) for their people.

Dr. Devareddy Narahari

Chapter 1

Introduction

More than 50% of the health status of all individuals is controlled by their lifestyle, food and food habits, because nutrition and health are closely related. Over the past few decades, several chronic diet-related and diet-influenced diseases have emerged, both in developed and in developing countries, due to consumption of unhealthy junk foods, excess calorie intake, faulty food habits and sedentary lifestyle behaviors. These poor eating habits, junk foods, faulty nutrition and lack of physical activity have a cumulative effect on the health status of individuals. By better nutrition, food habits and active lifestyle, many deadly diseases and disorders like CVD, some types of cancers, high blood pressure, IBS, obesity, acidity, type-2 diabetes, hyper-cholesterol, arthritis, liver and kidney disorders can be prevented or kept under control, without any medication.

The incidences of CVD, diabetes, cancer, hepatitis, bronchitis, nephritis, IBS, mental illness, lack of stamina, poor disease resistance, non-infectious chronic diseases and metabolic disorders are increasing at an alarming rate, year after year, all over the world—despite of medical advances. Until recently, the researchers, physicians, nutritionists and dieticians placed the blame for these increasing illnesses mostly on the food that was eaten—especially on the fats and cholesterol content in the food—ignoring many other real culprits.

Non-dietary causes like global changes in the environment, pollution, sedentary life style, lack of exercise, mental stress, tension, emotion, depression, broken families, and lack of cordial relationships at home, outside the home and at the workplace are contributing factors to a number of illnesses. As noted in Table-1-1, following, these non-dietary causes are responsible to the extent of 65-70% for most of the above diseases. Dietary causes that are responsible for these diseases include food adulteration, food additives, fast foods, refined foods, junk foods, street foods, food habits, imbalanced diets, and high calorie foods.

There is no doubt that diet plays a major role in the health status of any individual. A well-balanced diet of healthy food is essential for better health and a long life. However, there is lot of confusion and controversies about the right kind and nature of a well-balanced diet, even among nutritionists, researchers and doctors. Thousands of textbooks and research publications on nutrition, from various parts of the world, contradict each other, creating confusion among readers. Research done within a limited, short period, with small sample size, lack of meticulous data interpretation and correlation with other types of data, especially related to local conditions, will lead to wrong conclusions. Blindly following other countries recommendations, ignoring local situations, following old information and recommendations, ignoring the latest developments, will give contradicting and confusing results, also leading to wrong conclusions.

Conversely, all the latest scientific information collected from ACSH, ADA, AHA, AJCN, CDCS, CMFN, CNS, COMA, DHSS, EFSA, ENC, FAO, FDA FSIS, ICMR, ION, LPIMIC, LRCP, MRFIT, NAS, NCCAAHA, NCEPHLBI, NIN, NRC, RCPL, USDA, USDHHS, WHO, and various research stations and universities all over the world, over a prolonged period of time, are subjected to meta-analysis, comprehensive statistical and demographical interpretation, with logical and scientific reasoning. Based on these scientific, demographical and logical facts, linking this information meticulously with other scientific data, as well as by taking into account the local food habits and life style, food ingredients availability, food purchasing power, educational background, present local situations, religious beliefs, genetic make-up and socio-economic status, more valid conclusions can be drawn by the health authorities in each country, who can suggest true dietary guidelines and Recommended Daily Allowances (RDA) for their people.

For several decades, the health authorities around the globe have been recommending low fat, low cholesterol, low calorie and fiber-rich, balanced diets to control cardiovascular diseases, diabetes, IBS etc., but no significant improvement has been made in reducing the incidence of these diseases. On the other hand, the occurrence of these diseases is increasing alarmingly, year after year; especially in developing countries.

What is the reason? Where we have gone wrong?
If we probe critically and deeply into the causes of fast growing incidences of these diseases and in new emerging diseases, that have no benefits due to dietary restrictions—as mentioned above—we have to suspect some other dietary and non-dietary causes for all these ailments. They are not single causes, but many, and they are cumulative in nature, causing CVD, diabetes and other chronic diseases. They are not short-time, quick causes. They took several decades to worsen the health status. They will continue to worsen the health of many unless people recognize them and make necessary and possible changes.

What are these causes?
If we investigate the major changes that have taken place around the globe—in nature, population, environmental conditions, lifestyle, human behavior and overall food habits in the world—during the last few decades, we can observe the following significant changes, as shown in the Table-1-1 following.

Table-1-1: Global changes in the population, environment, food habits and lifestyle, during the past few decades, responsible for increased incidences of diabetes, CVD and other chronic diseases

Trait	Before 1950s	At present
Earth	More greenery, least pollution, provided ideal environment to the animals and plants for healthy living.	Humans becoming more and more selfish, creating excess pollution; over exploitation of the natural resources; excess use of fossil fuel, air conditioning, refrigeration, automobiles, factories, radiation due to holes in the ozone layer, etc., resulting in global warming.
Nature	Had enough untapped natural resources, especially green cover & rains, resulting in abundant availability of healthy, natural organic foods.	Most of the natural resources are fully tapped & exploited. Scarcity of safe air, water and food. Due to shortage of safe air, water and food, people are forced to breathe polluted air and consume unsafe water and food.
Population	World human population is below 3 billion, with plenty of fresh and safe food and water to share. No overcrowding & least competition.	Population has grown above 7.3 billion worldwide. Rapid population growth, especially in developing countries, is resulting in diminished resources, overcrowding, insufficient food and more competition.
Air pollution	Very few automobiles & industries, so less pollution. People are breathing fresh, uncontaminated air.	Automobiles & industries have gone up >100 times, so also pollution. People are forced to breathe highly polluted air having toxic gases, chemicals, carbon particles etc. throughout their life, resulting in several chronic and emerging diseases.

Food	Consuming all natural, safe and uncontaminated foods. Whole grains, no added preservatives, artificial colors, chemicals, flavoring agents, attractants & conditioners. No fast foods, refined foods, processed and further processed foods.	Due to work pressure, laziness to cook food at home, people are consuming more **junk foods**, mentioned in the previous column, having lots of sugar, hydrogenated fats (Vanaspathi /margarine etc.), refined flours (maida etc.), polished grains/pulses and many chemicals added as preservatives, coloring & flavoring agents to attract the customers. Added to these, present foods are having excess levels of harmful & carcinogenic pesticide residues.
Food additives	Very few or nil food additives are added to the food	Several carcinogenic and harmful food additives, in the name of food colors, flavors, preservatives, stabilizers, emulsifiers, anticaking, antifungal, binding agents are added to the foods, making the food a slow poison.
Drinking water	Have plenty of natural & safe drinking water from wells, rivers and springs. Such water will have several health promoting & immune-modulating ultra-trace elements and herbal extracts incorporated in the river water, while flowing.	Water scarcity leads to drinking of unsafe and polluted water by many. Even the treated water supplied by local bodies has a lot of chlorine, alum, activated carbon and other chemicals. The purified bottled water, due to constant contact with plastic, may have low levels of the chemicals in the plastic, especially carcinogenic, which may affect the consumers' health after several years of consumption.

Physical work & exercise	Due to lack of automation, people used to do lot of physical work like carrying heavy loads, laborious domestic works, various agriculture operations, plowing watering, washing, cleaning, cooking etc. resulting in perfect fitness and better health.	Due to excess use of automobiles, machinery, automatic domestic and office equipment and lethargy, there is very little physical work done. People find no time to do exercise like walking and are developing sedentary habits. Working night shifts and insufficient sleep. Added to these, refined and polished fast foods consumption, resulting in obesity, diabetes, cardiac and mental diseases.
Life style & behavior	Woke up early, completed daily routine in proper order, cooked and ate food at home, prepared from whole & near organic grains, seeds, vegetables & fruits, goes to work by walking or bicycle, goes to sleep early at night. Enjoys tension-free life.	Late from bread & to bed, rush to work by a vehicle, without completing daily routine, no exercise, no walking, eat outside junk fast foods made up of refined flours, sugar and chemical food additives. Suffers from a lot of stress, strain and tension at work, at home, as well as from other places due to growing unhealthy competition.
Relation-ship and friendship	Large families, each member will do some domestic work, share the responsibilities and maintain cordial relationships. Good neighbors, friends. All help reduce stress, depression, BP.	Broken & small families, mechanical life, no cordial relationship with family members, other relatives, office staff and neighbors. Friendship is skin deep. Have mechanical, depressed lifestyle.

Cosmetics	Very few cosmetics: soap, and face powder used by women.	Now the cosmetics industry is an ocean, and thousands of new cosmetics are continually dumped in the market. Many people spend more money on cosmetics than on health care and food. Most of these cosmetics are made up of chemicals which will affect the health of the users in the long run.
Electronic equipment	Only radio & land phone. No other electronic gadgets, no electro-magnetic waves, lasers from cell phones, computers and the internet.	Excess radiation from electronic gadgets, especially smart phones, Wi-Fi, internet, I-phones, I-pads, TV, computers etc. cause several diseases, interferes with brain function and pace maker in the heart.
Other factors	Enjoying near natural life, free from sound and light pollution. No mental disturbance.	Too much medication, drugs abuse & junk foods having several harmful chemicals are interfering with proper functioning of the heart, kidney, nervous system and increased incidence of cancer.

As shown in Table-1-1, non-dietary causes like global warming, radiation, pollution, sedentary habits, lifestyle, emotional stress, tension, depression, strained family and friendship relationships are the major causes of chronic and emerging diseases, rather than dietary causes. Besides the above major causes, extensive clinical and statistical studies have identified several individual orientated risk factors like age, gender (sex), smoking, drug abuse and diabetes are causing various heart, liver, lung and kidney disorders as well as cancer. To a greater extent, these non-dietary causes are responsible for these chronic diseases.

According to ADA,CNS,COMA,EFSA,ION,LRCP,NCCAAHA and other health authorities, there is no correlation between serum and dietary cholesterol levels, because the body can synthesize as much as 3000 mg of cholesterol per day. Moreover, as per WHO and FAO statistics, poor people from Afro-Asian countries, who are consuming less than 50 mg of cholesterol per day, and Eskimos, who are consuming more than 2000 mg of cholesterol per day, are having comparable serum cholesterol levels. But Eskimos are having lesser incidence of CVD, due to high HDL (good) cholesterol. Hence, they concluded that the serum and dietary cholesterol are independent. Therefore, many countries, including the USA, have removed the upper limit of 300 mg per day for dietary cholesterol in their RDA.

According to CDCS and CMFN, nutritionally poor and imbalanced diet, combined with physical inactivity, are the major causes of various ailments like obesity, cancer, diabetes, hypertension, hypercholesterolemia, arthritis, CVD and many more chronic disorders.

Excess calorie intake, especially from refined CHO, processed fast foods and junk foods like sweets, chips, French fries, samosas, snacks, bakery products made up of sugar, refined flour (maida etc.), butter and hydrogenated fats like margarine, shortening and /or vanaspathi (a hydrogenated vegetable fat used as a butter substitute in India and other countries) and artificial soft drinks loaded with harmful sugar—results in excess body weight, obesity, increased bad cholesterol and diabetes, which in turn leads to higher risk of cardio-vascular and other chronic diseases. Moreover, these fast foods are loaded with harmful trans-fatty acids, preservatives, colors, stabilizers, flavoring agents and other chemicals used to enhance the taste, flavor, crispiness, colour and eye appeal for foods which causes cancer, arthritis and other chronic diseases.

Sugar, refined flours and trans-fatty acids—rich hydrogenated fat, margarine, shortening and vanaspathi—are the worst foods and enemies of the mankind; they have to be avoided to safeguard your health. Trans fatty acids present in these junk foods act as **irritant,**

abrasive material and will injure the arterial wall, over which the cholesterol will be deposited; narrow the blood vessel and obstruct the free flow of blood; resulting in CVD and other health problems. If the arterial walls are intact and smooth, the cholesterol will flow freely and be soon excreted. Hence, there is no use of restricting the cholesterol, oil and fat intake, without restricting the total calorie intake and junk foods stuffed with sugar, refined flours, hydrogenated fats and many chemicals.

Moreover, unhealthy food habits and lifestyle are equally harmful for the health. Unhealthy food habits include:

- over eating
- fasting (fasting and feasting are equally harmful to the health)
- taking two or three heavy meals a day, instead of four to six small split meals
- exercising or sleeping soon after eating
- eating spoiled foods and/or imbalanced foods
- fast eating, eating too rapidly
- eating junk foods
- high calorie intake and many more

Dr. Dwight Lundell, a world famous cardiac surgeon, who has performed >5000 open heart surgeries and conducted extensive research for over a period of 25 years, also concluded that excess consumption of refined CHO rich fast foods is causing various health hazards, including CVD, diabetes, obesity, cancer and many more chronic diseases. Details of his investigations and speech are reported in the subsequent chapter. These unsafe foods include:

- sweets
- deep fried foods
- junk foods and sodas/soft drinks containing several hazardous chemicals in the name of food additives
- bakery products
- and frequently eating out (restaurant foods)

Most of the research/survey conducted on causes of diabetes, CVD and other chronic diseases are for a short duration, not exceeding five years, with a smaller sample size and confined to a smaller area. Hence, their findings are contradicting to each other and not reliable, creating confusion among health authorities and the public. On the other hand, the changes and observations reported in the above Table-1-1 are for over a period of more than six decades, covering the entire world; therefore, these observations are more authenticated and realistic. It clearly indicates that multi-various factors—mostly non-dietary factors—are responsible for the present day health situation. These continuing global changes over decades—and even for centuries—have not only worsened the health status of the people gradually; they have also resulted in the introduction of new emerging diseases and the weakening of immunity systems. However, our society cannot go back to pre-1950 situation to reduce the incidences of several chronic and emerging diseases, but we can make certain healthy changes:

- walking/getting sufficient exercise
- eating home-made foods made up of whole grains, multiple vegetables and fruits
- getting sufficient sleep
- minimizing stress by doing yoga, meditation, breathing exercises, maintaining cordial family relationships, friendly work-related atmosphere, positive thinking, optimistic behavior, having good relationships with family friends and neighbors.
- avoid smoking

Prima-facie the question of excess saturated fat or even oil consumption in India and other developing countries does not arise; because **India is in the bottom of the table in the per capita total lipid (oil + fat) consumption in the world**, as per the demography of FAO, USDA and NIN, which is reported in detail in subsequent chapters. Now many health authorities in many countries are recommending 25-30 % of the total calories from lipids in their diet. For example, if a person needs 2000 Kcal./day, 25-30 % of it : 500 -

600 Kcal. must come from lipids. At the rate of 9 Kcal /g of lipid, a minimum of 500 /600÷9: 55.5 to 66.7 or average 60 g lipids are needed per day. In developed countries, the food calories of lipid origin are 35 to 40% of total calories consumed. The health authorities in these countries are suggesting to reduce it to 25 -30% levels. **The reverse is true in India**. NIN's (2011) RDA for Indians, for visible oil /fat consumption, is just 30 g, which is far lower (almost half) than the RDA by many other countries; but actually, the actual consumption of visible lipids by an average Indian is about 12 g (40% of low RDA) only.

Dr. Mark Hyman (2016), a popular physician cum nutritionist in USA in TV shows, is stating **"Eat Fat and get Thin"**— provided that the total calorie intake/day is within the RDA for the individuals, based on their physical activity and body weight. Based on several studies in various universities, the ADA, AHA and USDA have withdrawn the upper limit for egg consumption and dietary cholesterol levels and increased the total SFA levels from 10 to 12% of total calories.

So, people in developing countries are actually suffering from deficiency of total lipids EFA-PUFA fat-soluble vitamins (especially vitamin A & E) and proteins, in comparison to excess consumption in many developed countries. Hence, dieticians in developing countries have to recommend to decrease CHO and total calories and increase the calories of lipid origin to at least 25 % of total calories.** Ignoring these facts, some health authorities in developing countries are still recommending outdated and harmful low fat and low cholesterol diets to their customers, resulting in consumption of high CHO (starchy & sugary) foods, which will be converted to body fat and cause more harm.

Fundamentals of biochemistry and metabolism say that the three major nutrients—carbohydrates-CHO (starch & sugars), lipids (fats & oils) and proteins—are the sources of energy (calories) to the body. They are interconvertible in the body. CHO are the first choice as body fuel (energy). If it is deficient, fats will be utilized for energy purpose, and finally the protein. Excess of one of these three will be converted to the other which is deficient, or converted to the body fat. This synthesized body fat is mainly the saturated fatty acid, stearic acid, because the body cannot synthesize essential poly-unsaturated fatty acids (PUFA).

Cholesterol is the mother of all hormones secreted in the body: anti-ageing hormone, Vitamin-D, active constituent of nervous tissue, bile and many other essential secretions/products in the body. Hence, without cholesterol there is no life. It has been well established beyond any doubt that cholesterol is essential to perform various body functions (discussed in detail in another Chapter), but it is not dietary essential because our body can synthesize as much as 3000 mg of cholesterol per day (endogenous). If cholesterol is available in the food, its biosynthesis will be proportionately reduced by feedback mechanism. In a healthy person, the sum of endogenous and exogenous cholesterol for a given period is more or less constant.

Moreover, the dietary cholesterol absorption rate varies from 15 to 71% (average 40%) and is inversely proportional to the level of cholesterol in the food. **A healthy vegan, who consume '0' cholesterol, will have normal serum cholesterol levels, due to sufficient cholesterol biosynthesis. On the other hand, Eskimos, who consume the highest dietary cholesterol per day (>2000 mg/day), will also have normal serum cholesterol levels, due to low biosynthesis or quick excretion of it. Hence, dietary cholesterol plays no role on serum cholesterol levels, and these two are independent entities. Based on these reliable repeated findings over several decades, the American Dietetic Association (ADA) lifted the upper ceiling of 300 mg cholesterol per day in 2014, and now there is no restriction on cholesterol consumption. Many other countries also are not prescribing any upper limit for cholesterol consumption, but still our NIN is advising to restrict the cholesterol intake to less than 200 mg/day. In fact, the average dietary cholesterol consumption in India is a meagre 60 mg/day, which is one of the lowest in the world. Then what is the necessity for further reduction of**

cholesterol intake, and how it is going to improve the health of individuals?

Unfortunately, due to lack of sufficient "in-depth research" in developing countries, their dieticians, nutritionists and physicians are simply adapting the recommendations of developed countries to their people, ignoring the existing actual local situations into account. Low protein, low lipid and excess CHO diet in the developing countries make many people diabetic at an early age. **Therefore, the recommendations must be to take more lipids (25-30% calories, instead of 17%) and proteins (13 % calories, instead of 10%) and consume lesser CHO (<60 % instead of 73% calories).**

Moreover, our health authorities are advising our people to avoid or minimize the consumption of lipids, cholesterol, meats and eggs (good quality protein), even though no such negative advice is given in any other country where the meat consumptions are 10 to 100 times higher and the egg consumption is 5 to 6 times higher than in India. **India is the best example for wrongful dietary advice**. In India, the total red meat and chicken meat consumptions are 5.1 and 2.2 kg, respectively, and ranks among the bottom most 5% in meat eating in the world. Many countries are recommending a minimum of 30 to 50 g of meat (preferably lean meat from chicken and fish) per person per day, whereas in India it is <14 g/day, resulting in protein deficiency. Similarly, our per-capita consumption of 55 eggs per annum is a meagre 30 % of the WHO's minimum recommended levels of 183 eggs (1/2 egg/day) and no upper limit is prescribed for egg consumption. Our NIN is also recommending 3 eggs per week. The real egg consumption in India is 57, which is one of the lowest in the world, ranking among the bottom 10%. This low egg consumption in India is not due to poverty (the egg prices in India are comparable with that of many vegetables and fruits); it is due to religious taboos, ignorance and misguidance by the health authorities.

In a healthy diet, at least 1/3rd of total protein must be of animal origin, like milk, meat and eggs, because animal proteins have balanced amino acid profile and higher biological value than

26

vegetable protein. Such extremely low consumption of lipids and proteins has resulted in protein and PUFA deficiency. This also leads to excess consumption of CHO, resulting in more incidences of diabetes and also CVD (Lundell, 2015). As per the data available in 2015 from different authenticated sources like WHO, India has the fastest growing incidence of diabetes in the world. About 18.5% of the world's diabetics are in India. The actual figure must be higher than this, because many millions of poor diabetic patients in rural areas are not included in this list. The details are discussed in the subsequent chapters.

Now many nutritionists in the USA, Europe, Mexico, China, Japan and many other developed countries are recommending two eggs for breakfast; which will give satiety, supply high biological value balanced nutrients, and at the same time supply low calories of non-CHO origin (140 Kcal. from 2 eggs) for weight loss and better health. Meat, egg, cholesterol, fat and saturated fat consumption in India is one of the lowest in the world, (more details in subsequent chapters). Under such circumstances, there is no logic in advising our people to reduce their cholesterol, lipid, meat and egg consumption. Such false recommendations will only produce negative results like excess CHO consumption and diabetes. So we have to follow a different dietary strategy, suitable for us, based on the present facts and not borrowed from other countries where the situations are different.

Added to these false interpretations and wrong recommendations, the vegans and animal welfare activists are creating panic in the minds of the public and even confusing the physicians, dieticians and nutritionists with the intention of converting the entire society as vegetarians. They are a very strong, affluent and influential lobby. If their argument is correct, all of them must be free from any CVD, cholesterol and live longer. However, available authenticated statistical data from various sources and many countries have indicated that both vegetarians and non-vegetarians are equally susceptible to CVD and hyper cholesterol. Moreover, higher incidence of Alzheimer's, dementia, depression and other nervous disorders are recorded among vegans, due to deficiency of vitamin B12, DHA and EPA, in their diets.

Certain essential nutrients like Vitamin B12, D3, carnosine, creatine, EPA, DHA, taurine, and many essential amino acids, are either deficient or absent in plant tissues; for these essential nutrients, we have to depend on foods of animal origin. Humans are born omnivorous, with canine teeth. The first profession known to humans is hunting, followed by agriculture. Both plants and animals are living things created by God and liked by God equally. Humans must depend on plants and animals for their food and other needs. We should not harm plants and animals for fun and other selfish needs; we should harvest them only for food; and that, too, should be done in a humane way. This is not a debate for vegetarianism vs. non-vegetarianism, only to bring to light the latest facts and figures. The choice is left to the physicians, dieticians and the public, based on the facts.

Chapter 2

What Really Causes CVD & Other Chronic Diseases?

Multiple factors are responsible for these diseases, including genetic make-up of the individuals, race, diet and dietary habits, environmental pollution, physical activity, life style, emotional stress, depression and tension, smoking, drug abuse, positive/negative attitudes, presence of other diseases, obesity and many more. All these causes will not lead to CVD and other heart diseases overnight; it will take several years or even decades for these diseases to appear. Additional causes for these diseases are added every year, and they vary from place to place.

Dr. Dwight Lundell is a world-renowned heart surgeon and the past Chief of Staff and Chief of Surgery at Banner Heart Hospital, Mesa, AZ. His private practice, Cardiac Care Center, was in Mesa, AZ. Recently Dr. Lundell left surgery to focus on the nutritional treatment of heart disease. He is the founder of Healthy Humans Foundation, which promotes human health, with a focus on helping large corporations promote wellness. He is also the author of *The Cure for Heart Disease* and *The Great Cholesterol Lie*. He spoke on *What Really Causes Heart Diseases* on January 21, 2015.

We physicians, with all our training, knowledge and authority, often acquire a rather large ego that tends to make it difficult to admit we are wrong. So, here it is. I freely admit to being wrong. As a heart surgeon with 25 years' experience, having performed over 5,000 open-heart surgeries, today is my day to right the wrong with medical and scientific facts.

I have trained for many years along with other prominent physicians labelled as "opinion makers." Bombarded with scientific literature, continually attending education seminars, we opinion makers insisted heart disease resulted from the simple fact of elevated blood cholesterol. The only accepted therapy was prescribing medications to lower cholesterol and a diet that severely restricted fat intake. The latter, we insisted, would lower cholesterol and heart disease. Deviations from these recommendations were considered heresy and could quite possibly result in malpractice.

It Is Not Working!
These recommendations are no longer scientifically or morally defensible. The discovery a few years ago that **inflammation in the artery wall is the real cause of heart disease** is slowly leading to a paradigm shift in how heart disease and other chronic ailments will be treated. **The long-established false dietary recommendations have created epidemics of obesity and diabetes**, the consequences of which dwarf any historical plague in terms of mortality, human suffering and dire economic consequences. Despite the fact that 25% of the population takes expensive statin medications, and we have reduced the fat content of our diets, more Americans will die this year of heart disease than ever before. Statistics from the **American Heart Association** show that 75 million Americans currently suffer from heart disease, 20 million have diabetes and 57 million have pre-diabetes. These disorders are affecting younger and younger people in greater numbers every year.

In many developing Afro-Asian countries, the problem is still worse because we are simply copying the dietary recommendations of the USA and other developed countries, where the dietary pattern, food habits and other non-dietary factors varies. For example, the problem in developed countries is excess calorie intake, especially from lipids (fats/oils) origin, which accounts for nearly 40 % of total calories. Hence, the dieticians and doctors there are advising people to reduce fat calories from 40 % to 25-30 %. The condition in developing countries is entirely different, where the total calories of lipid origin are less than 20% (12 % in India). In such case, if the doctors advise to reduce fat calories further, it will lead to over consumption of calories of CHO (starch and sugars) origin (>75% calories of CHO origin, instead of <60%), resulting in more and more diabetes cases.

Another leading cardiologist, Dr. Arash Bereliani (2016), after several years of study has concluded that the first step leading to CVD is inflammation (irritation) of the arterial wall. This inflammation is caused by any irritant material, like oxidizing agents, trans-fatty acids, and free radicals, which are formed due to processing and further processing of foods, such as deep frying for a long time, hydrogenation, rancidity, improper storage, prolonged storage and addition of several food additives (chemicals) having irritant properties. These irritant substances act as abrasive material (like sand paper) and damage the arterial walls, over which the cholesterol, waxy materials and blood clots will be deposited.

Simply stated, that without inflammation being present in the artery, there is no way that cholesterol would accumulate in the wall of the blood vessel and cause heart disease and strokes. Without inflammation, cholesterol would move freely throughout the artery as nature intended. It is the inflammation that causes cholesterol to become trapped. Inflammation is not complicated—it is quite simply your body's natural defense to a foreign invader such as a bacteria, toxin or virus. The cycle of inflammation is perfect in how it protects your body from these bacterial and viral invaders. However, if we chronically expose the body to injury by toxins or foods the human body was never designed to process, a condition occurs called chronic inflammation. Chronic inflammation is just as harmful as acute inflammation. What thoughtful person would willfully expose himself repeatedly to foods or other substances that are known to cause injury to the body and blood vessels? Well, smokers perhaps, but at least they made that choice willfully.

The rest of us have simply followed the recommended mainstream diet that is low in fat and high in polyunsaturated fats and carbohydrates, not knowing that we were causing repeated injury to our blood vessels. This repeated injury creates chronic inflammation, leading to heart disease, stroke, diabetes and obesity.

Let me repeat that: The injury and inflammation in our blood vessels is caused by the low fat diet recommended for years by mainstream medicine. What are the biggest culprits of chronic inflammation? Quite simply, chronic consumption of simple, highly processed carbohydrates (sugar, flour and all the products made from them, like bakery products and sweets) will increase blood sugar levels beyond the threshold levels of the tissues. Trans-fatty acids, like elaidic and vaccinic acid are produced during repeated prolonged boiling of oils rich in omega-6 PUFA (linoleic acid) like soybean, corn, sunflower and safflower oils, for continuous frying in restaurants—especially French fries and chips. During this over boiling process, the fatty acid-linoleic acid (also called *cis,* fatty acid) will transform into trans-fatty acids. Similarly, during hydrogenation process for production of hydrogenated fats (Vanaspathi), margarines etc., trans-fatty acids are formed. Continuous consumption of these trans-fatty acids—rich foods like margarine, French fries, chips and other fried foods—will increase the oxidative trans-fatty acid levels in the blood; these high levels will act as abrasive material, cause injury, inflammation and abrasions to the arterial walls. The cholesterol and other waxy substances will stick to the abrasive (damaged) arterial walls, forming plaques, which will block the free flow of blood in the arteries, resulting in CVD. If there is no damage to the arterial walls, the cholesterol will flow freely in the blood vessels.

Take a moment to visualize rubbing a stiff brush repeatedly over soft skin until it becomes quite red and nearly bleeding. You kept this up several times a day, every day for five years. If you could tolerate this painful brushing, you would have a bleeding, swollen infected area that became worse with each repeated injury. This is a good way to visualize the inflammatory process that could be going on in your body right now.

Regardless of where the inflammatory process occurs, externally or internally, it is the same. I have peered inside thousands upon thousands of arteries. A diseased artery looks as if someone took a brush and scrubbed repeatedly against its wall. Several times a day, every day, the foods we eat create small injuries compounding into more injuries, causing the body to respond continuously and appropriately with inflammation.

While we savor the tantalizing taste of a sweet roll, our bodies respond alarmingly, as if a foreign invader has arrived, declaring war. Foods loaded with sugars and simple carbohydrates, or processed with trans-fatty acids for long shelf life, have been the mainstay of the American diet for six decades. These foods have been slowly poisoning everyone.

How does eating a simple sweet roll create a cascade of inflammation to make you sick?

Imagine spilling syrup on your computer keyboard and you have a visual of what occurs inside the cell. When we consume simple carbohydrates such as sugar, blood sugar rises rapidly. In response, your pancreas secretes insulin, whose primary purpose is to drive sugar into each cell where it is stored for energy. If the cell is full and does not need glucose, it is rejected to avoid extra sugar gumming up the works. When your full cells reject the extra glucose, blood sugar rises, producing more insulin, and the glucose converts to stored fat.

What does all this have to do with inflammation?

Blood sugar is controlled in a very narrow range. Extra sugar molecules attach to a variety of proteins that in turn injure the blood vessel wall. This repeated injury to the blood vessel wall sets off inflammation. When you spike your blood sugar level several times a day, every day, it is exactly like taking sandpaper to the inside of your delicate blood vessels. While you may not be able to see it, rest assured it is there. I saw it in over 5,000 surgical patients, spanning

25 years, who all shared one common denominator-- **inflammation in their arteries.**

Let's get back to the sweet roll.
That innocent looking goody not only contains sugars, it is baked in one of many omega-6 oils such as soybean or trans-fatty-acid-rich hydrogenated fat or margarine. Chips and fries are soaked in soybean oil; processed foods are manufactured with omega-6 oils for longer shelf life. While omega-6's are essential—they are part of every cell membrane controlling what goes in and out of the cell— they must be in the correct balance with omega-3's (omega-6: 3 ::6:1 ratio). If the balance shifts by consuming excessive omega-6, the cell membrane produces chemicals called **cytokines** that directly cause inflammation.

Today's mainstream American diet has produced an extreme imbalance of these two fats. The ratio of imbalance ranges from 15:1 to as high as 30:1 in favor of omega-6. That's a tremendous amount of **cytokines** causing inflammation. In today's food environment, a 3:1 ratio would be optimal and healthy.

To make matters worse, the excess weight you are carrying from eating these foods creates overloaded fat cells that pour out large quantities of **pro-inflammatory chemicals** that add to the injury caused by having high blood sugar. The process that began with a sweet roll turns into a vicious cycle over time that creates heart disease, high blood pressure, diabetes and finally, Alzheimer's disease, as the inflammatory process continues unabated. There is no escaping the fact that the more we consume prepared and processed foods, the more we trip the inflammation switch little by little each day. The human body cannot process, nor was it designed to consume, foods packed with sugars and soaked in omega-6 oils.

There is but one answer to quieting inflammation, and that is returning to foods closer to their natural state. To build muscle, eat more protein. Choose carbohydrates that are very complex, such as unpolished bran-rich whole grains and fresh colorful fruits and vegetables. Cut down on or eliminate inflammation causing foods rich in trans-fatty acids like hydrogenated fats, repeatedly boiled oils, French fries and all deep fried items from restaurants, sugars, refined flours and processed junk foods that are made from them.

Replace corn, sunflower and safflower oils with olive, soybean, sesame, peanut or canola oils. Even grass fed cows' butter/ghee and chicken fat/oil, can be used for cooking. Animal fats containing less than 20% omega-6 are much less likely to cause inflammation than the supposedly healthy oils labelled polyunsaturated. Forget the "science" that has been drummed into your head for decades. The science that saturated fat alone causes heart disease is non-existent. The science that saturated fat raises blood cholesterol is also very weak. Since we now know that cholesterol is not the cause of heart disease, the concern about saturated fat is even more absurd today.

The cholesterol theory led to the no-fat, low-fat recommendations that in turn created the very foods now causing an epidemic of inflammation. Mainstream medicine made a terrible mistake when it advised people to avoid saturated fat in favor of foods high in omega-6 PUFA. We now have an epidemic of arterial inflammation leading to heart disease and other silent killers.

What you can do is choose whole foods available >60 years back, **prepared at home** by your **grandmother** (foods eaten prior to 1950). As far as possible consume **homemade foods** and avoid outside junk foods from supermarkets and restaurants, from street restaurants to seven star hotels. These foods are made more attractive, tasty, with better flavor and color by adding various chemicals, preservatives,, coloring and flavoring agents, by deep-frying in trans-fatty acids, rich margarine, vanaspathi and over-boiled oils. Avoid modern processed-refined-junk-fast foods, made up of refined CHO + sugars + several harmful food additives—especially sweetened sodas. By eliminating inflammatory junk foods and adding essential nutrients from fresh, unprocessed whole grains, vegetables and fruits, you can reverse years of damages caused in your arteries and throughout your body by these junk foods.

Chapter 3

Myths and Facts in Nutrition

There are more **myths** than facts in nutrition and food information, creating confusion and a fear complex among the public. Moreover, many web sites, consultants and pharmaceuticals often give wrong and confusing information about foods for their commercial gains. Some of the myths are discussed below. Many are giving false suggestions based on old textbook information, not updating their technical information, and are ignoring the fundamentals of biochemistry, basal metabolism, different food practices in different places and their effects on the local population in the long run and demography.

Myths	Facts
Non-vegetarian foods will increase serum cholesterol & risk of cardio-vascular diseases (CVD)	If this statement is true, then developed countries, where the per capita consumption of non-vegetarian foods is 20-30 times higher than in poor Afro-Asian countries (actual consumption in many countries are shown in other chapters), must have 20-30 times more incidence of CVD; but in reality, they are having lesser incidences, indicating that non-vegetarian foods are as safe as vegetarian foods. First of all, it has been well established by several health authorities that **there is no correlation between dietary and serum cholesterol levels and that these two are independent entities**. More than 40 % of Indians are vegetarians; but the incidence of CVD

	and diabetes are equally distributed among vegetarians and non-vegetarians. Excess calorie intake, especially of sugar and refined carbohydrates origin, with low protein and essential fatty acids, combined with sedentary lifestyle, are high risk factors for CVD and diabetes. Fish is always good for better health due to its essential heart friendly omega-3 PUFA (EPA & DHA) and amino acids rich in high quality protein. Similarly, lean and tender chicken meat, without skin, has less than 4% fat and insignificant cholesterol (just like milk), but supplies high quality protein. Chicken and egg fats are more unsaturated than milk fat (butter). Diabetics need more protein and lipids and less CHO. Hence, a 3:1 mixture of vegetarian and non-vegetarian foods is more suitable for all, especially diabetics, children, pregnant women, mothers giving breast milk, and old and sick persons.
Cholesterol is a dangerous, unwanted and harmful substance	In fact, cholesterol is an essential substance for all animals, including humans. About 0.2% of our body weight is cholesterol. It is the **mother of all hormones** in our body, without which we cannot survive. It is an essential component of all nervous tissues, bile, Vit-D3, most of the hormones, and plays a major role in reproduction and metabolism. The body can synthesize enough cholesterol to perform the above functions if there is no or insufficient dietary cholesterol. **Therefore, ADA & AHA has recently removed the upper limit for dietary cholesterol level.**
Cholesterol consumption will increase serum LDL (bad) cholesterol. Hence,	As per WHO, ADA, USDA reports, **Eskimos, who are consuming the highest cholesterol/day (>2000 mg) have safe serum cholesterol levels and lesser incidence of CVD, compared to low economy Afro-Asians, whose daily cholesterol consumption is as low as 50 mg/day.** Even vegans, who consume

avoid cholesterol rich foods.	"nil" cholesterol, will have enough or excess cholesterol in the body, compared to others, due to cholesterol biosynthesis. Our body can synthesize as much as 3000 mg of cholesterol per day. High serum cholesterol is due to either failure in the body mechanism of controlling the cholesterol synthesis or failure in its excretion mechanism, which in turn is due to several causes for many decades. It is mainly due to **many non-dietary factors**, like heredity, obesity, pollution, sedentary lifestyle, age, smoking, gender, tension, emotional stress; **several medical conditions** like diabetes, obesity, abrasion to the arterial walls, hypothyroidism, constipation, chronic liver and renal (kidney) disorders, hormonal imbalance; **and drugs** like steroids and progesterone (birth control pills), as explained in other chapters. Dietary causes are relatively less, compared to non-dietary causes. People are eating fast foods and **junk foods** rich in sugars, refined flour, margarine, vanaspathi and trans-fatty acids, present in sweets, bakery products, French fries, chips and other junk foods; are having excess calorie and CHO consumption, are over eating, and have an imbalanced diet.
Vegetarian foods are good for health	No doubt vegetarian foods, mainly fresh mixed fruits, vegetables—especially green leafy vegetables—and whole unpolished/unrefined grains and pulses are good for health, provided they are free from pesticides, herbicides and other harmful chemicals used during agriculture and processing. However, continuous consumption of junk vegetarian foods having high levels of sugar, refined CHO, margarine, vanaspathi, high calorie junk foods are cholesterol-genic and diabeto-genic. Moreover, in general all vegetarian foods are deficient in many essential nutrients like amino acids, Vit-B12, D3, choline, creatinine, taurine, EPA and DHA. A

	really balanced food is one having a right combination of both vegetarian and non-vegetarian foods of different varieties, in 3:1 ratio. In fact, foods of animal origin, especially eggs, chicken and fish are very good anti-diabetic foods, due to zero calories from CHO, and contain essential fatty acids and high biological value protein.
Fasting is good for health	Fasting is good during stomach upset and indigestion, but not for diabetic and other conditions. It is not suitable for weight control. So **both fasting and feasting are not good for health.** It is especially true for diabetics. Diabetics must eat small quantities of food rich in complex CHO, rich in fiber and essential fatty acids and amino acids at frequent intervals, preferably 5 or 6 times a day, to maintain near normal blood sugar levels. They must snack in between breakfast, lunch, dinner and before going to bed. Now dieticians in developed countries are recommending a heavy breakfast (because no food is taken for the past 12 hours—overnight), a light lunch and moderate dinner for healthy living. On health grounds, breakfast shall not be skipped.
Low fat foods are good for health	Low fat foods are usually deficient in essential fatty acids and fat-soluble vitamins. They are especially not suitable for growing children and diabetics. Research teams in many universities in the USA have concluded that whole milk is more suitable for growing children and diabetics than low fat or skimmed milk. Unlike CHO, lipids will release energy slowly and have very low glycemic index; hence, they are good for diabetics. In India, dieticians are still recommending low fat foods, copying the recommendations of developed countries and ignoring the local situations. Western countries are recommending to their people to reduce the fat calories from 40 % to 30 % and increase calories of CHO origin, to at least 55 %. Dr. Mark Hyman (2016), USA, is recommending, "**Eat Fat**

	& Get Thin." On the other hand, in our country, the existing calorie intake from lipids and CHO are 17 and 73%, respectively. Hence, for better health, Indians have to increase their calories of lipid origin from 17 to 25-30% and reduce the calories of CHO origin from 73 to <60%.
Harmful antibiotics and drug residues are present in the meat.	As per WHO, USDA, FAO and government regulations, poultry farmers are either feeding their birds with antibiotic-free feed or following antibiotics withdrawal from feeds 10 days before processing of the birds so that there will not be any drug residues left in the egg and meat, or may be present within the safe permissible levels. In case of other meat animals, they are fed only by grazing in the fields and there is no scientific feeding, so the question of drug residues will not arise. Moreover, the meat consumption in poor Afro-Asian countries is one of the lowest in the world, which is not even 5% of the meat consumed in developed countries. Hence, at this low consumption of meat and eggs, it will not affect the health, even if antibiotic residues are present above the permissible levels. Furthermore, compared to the antibiotic residues, the pesticides/insecticides/herbicides residues in vegetables and fruits are more dangerous to the human health.
Hormones are present in meat, which makes girls come to puberty early and affects the health of others.	First of all, hormones are very expensive and costlier than the chicken. Therefore, it is not economical to use in poultry production in any part of the world. In the case of beef cattle, growth hormones are used in beef producing countries like Argentina, Brazil, USA etc. But they, too, are withdrawing well in advance before slaughter. In poor countries, there is no scientific beef production and hormones are not at all used. In case of milk animals, some cattle owners are illegally (not permitted) injecting oxytocin hormone to the animal, prior to milking, for complete evacuation of the milk from the

	udder. Moreover, hormones are denatured during cooking and in the digestive tack. As a result, there are no negative results to the consumers, but they affect animal health. Since animal protein is a better protein than vegetable protein, regular consumption of lean meat provides better health and faster growth rate in children, which was mistaken as the effect of hormones.
Animal proteins causes cancer	If animal proteins are causing cancer, the incidence of cancer in developed countries, where the per capita consumption of non-vegetarian foods is 20-30 times more than in India, must be 20-30 times more than in India; but in reality, there are no such variations, indicating that non-vegetarian foods are as safe as vegetarian foods. However, factory made, further processed, ready-to-eat red meat products, as well as other junk foods like soft drinks, French fries, bakery products and sweets etc. having various food additives, are harmful for health if there is no sufficient fiber in the diet. In fact, **egg albumen prevents various types of gastro-intestinal cancers, breast cancer etc.**
Refined junk foods, like sweets, cakes, cookies, burgers, French fries, chips and other deep fried restaurant foods, sodas etc. having several harmful **food**	Yes, continuous consumption of junk foods are partly responsible for various chronic diseases like CVD, diabetes, etc., but they are not solely responsible, as stated in other chapters. Food habits like consuming an imbalanced diet, over eating, untimely eating, outside restaurant foods instead of homemade foods, taking fruits along with main food and chronic alcoholism also contributes to these diseases to some extent. Besides dietary causes, non-dietary causes like genetic background, lack of exercise, sedentary habits, modern lifestyle, stress, tension, emotions, smoking, pollution of all kinds, insufficient sleep, depression and lack of family relationships are the major contributing factors to these diseases.

additives (chemicals) causes various chronic diseases like CVD, cancer, diabetes, etc.	
Artificial sweeteners are acceptable for diabetics	This is only a self-satisfying and miss-guiding statement. Even though the artificial sweeteners like saccharine, aspartame, neotame, Ace-K, advantame, cyclamate, stevia, sucralose etc. are calorie free, they have several side effects, including carcinogenic effect. Hence, they are not advisable. It is better to avoid both artificial sweeteners as well as calorie-rich sugars and develop taste for bitter coffee, tea and other beverages.

Chapter 4

How Much Water Do You Need Daily?

Water is a major and most important nutrient for all living beings on earth, because they are mostly made up of water. About two-thirds of the human body is nothing but water. Therefore, water is the most important and abundantly required nutrient for all living beings. Women have relatively lower water than men because they have a higher proportion of body fat. The same rule applies to people who are overweight or obese. Growing children and pregnant /lactating women will have an increased proportion of water in their body. On the other hand, old persons will have a lesser proportion of water in their body.

Functions of water:

1. Water is the media in which our body exists, so all bio-chemical functions in the body are performed in the water media.

2. Water is essential for all body cells to perform various bio-chemical and metabolic reactions properly.

3. Water, as a major part of blood, will transport all nutrients and oxygen to all tissues and cells in the body.

4. Similarly, water will remove all waste toxic materials from the body through urine, sweat, respiration (vapor loss), stools, sneezing, coughing and other fluid loss.

5. Water is involved in thermoregulatory mechanism and thereby regulates body temperature.

Water sources:
The body obtains water primarily by absorbing it from the digestive tract. This water is called exogenous (outside) water, which comes from both the food we eat as well as the water and fluids we drink. Additionally, some amount of water is produced by the body during metabolism, called **metabolic water or indigenous water**.

Ultimately, the body will obtain water from the following:

   i. water and fluids we consume

   ii. from foods we eat and

   iii. metabolic water produced in the body.

Metabolic water:
During breakdown (oxidation, using oxygen in the blood) of CHO, proteins and lipids in the tissues for energy release, 6 molecules of water and 6 molecules of carbon dioxide will be released as follows:

$$C_6 H_{12} O_6 + 6O_2 = 6 CO_2 + 6H_2O + \text{energy released}$$

This CO_2 will be transported into the lungs through blood for excretion through exhaled air. During oxidation of 100 g of CHO, lipids and proteins in the body for energy release, 55 g, 110 g and 41.3 g of water is produced, respectively. As such 350 to 400 ml (1 ml=1 g) of metabolic water is produced daily in the body, depending on the energy requirement and the nature of food consumed. This metabolic water accounts for 8-10% of the daily water requirement.

Water requirement:
There is lot of confusion regarding the water requirement of persons. Many dieticians and doctors recommend a fixed amount and schedule of water intake per day, like 1-2 cups of water soon after waking up from bed, 1 cup before each meal and little or no water during or after food. This fixed quantity of water consumption not correct, because the water requirement varies with individuals, based on their age, type of food consumed, extent of water in the foods consumed, environmental temperature, relative humidity,

extent of physical activity, sweating nature, urinary output, diseases like diarrhea, dysentery and many more factors.

In 2004 the Food and Nutrition Board (FNB) has recommended a water intake of about 1.5 ml/kcal of energy consumed/day. As such, a person consuming 2000 kcal /day needs 3 liters (3000 ml) of water/day. Therefore, based on various factors influencing the water requirement, the daily water requirement of persons varies from 3 to 4 liters per day, of which nearly 8-10% is from metabolic water, 20-25% from foods and the remaining 65-72% (2-3 liters) is from drinking water and other fluids.

- More drinking water has to be consumed if the food we eat is dry or semi-dry, and vice-versa is also true. Liquid foods taken, like milk, soup, porridge, fruit juice lessens the drinking water requirement.

- More drinking water has to be consumed with protein rich foods (due to lesser metabolic water), salt, fiber rich foods and deep fried foods. Less water is needed for CHO rich and steam-cooked foods.

- During high environmental temperatures and during exercise, there will be more sweating, resulting in water loss, which has to be replaced by more water intake.

- Those who urinate more quantity and frequently, such as diabetics, poly-urea, due to various reasons, have to replace the water loss to prevent dehydration.

- Persons suffering from diarrhea, a cold with lot of nasal discharge, vomiting, poly urea, poly-dipsia, dysentery, blood loss and any fluid loss have to rehydrate themselves by consuming more water.

- **Whenever we feel thirsty, we have to consume sufficient water to the extent of overcoming the thirst, irrespective of all other factors.** Never ignore thrust and dehydration.

The water intake must balance the water loss. To maintain water balance and to protect against dehydration, prevent the development of kidney stones and other medical problems, healthy adults should drink 2 to 3 liters of water/fluids a day, depending on the water in the food consumed, sweating, outside temperature, exercise and physical work, urinary loss and other fluid loses.

Body water loss:

If your body loses 1% water, you feel thirsty, and if your body loses 2% water, you suffer from severe dehydration, which is very dangerous. Blood becomes thicker. The brain may not get enough blood, resulting in fainting. Both excess and lesser water consumption are not good for health. But drinking excess water is less dangerous than drinking insufficient water, because excreting excess water is much easier for the body than conserving water. However, when the kidneys are functioning normally, the body can handle wide variations in fluid intake.

The body loses water primarily by excreting it through urine from the kidneys. Depending on the body's needs, the kidneys may excrete less than a pint to more than a gallon of urine a day. Another 600 ml to one liter of water is lost daily as sweat and in exhaled air through the lungs. Profuse sweating due to vigorous exercise, hot weather, or due to high body temperature, can dramatically increase the amount of water lost through evaporation. Less than 300 ml of water is excreted through stools. However, prolonged vomiting or severe diarrhea can result in the loss of electrolytes and 2-3 liters or more water a day. In such case, the affected person needs rehydration, along with electrolytes.

Drinking a good amount of water could lower your risk of a heart attack. A six-year study published in the *American Journal of Epidemiology* found that people who drank more than five glasses of water a day were 41 % less likely to die from a heart attack than those who drank less than two glasses of water. Moreover, drinking all that water may reduce the risk of cancer as well. Research showed that staying hydrated can reduce the risk of colon cancer by 45 %, bladder cancer by 50 % and possibly reduce breast cancer risk also. The qualities of safe drinking water is mentioned in **Table-4.1** following.

Serial No.	Substance	Maximum permissible level (ppm)	Desirable level (ppm)
1	Total dissolved solids	2000	500
2	Salinity	500	300
3	Total alkalinity	200	100
4	Total hardness	600	300
5	PH	6.0 – 8.0	6.8 – 7.2
6	Calcium	200	75
7	Magnesium	100	30
8	Sodium	400	50
9	Chloride	400	100
10	Bicarbonate	400	100
11	Sulphate	400	125
12	Fluoride	1.5	1
13	Nitrate	50	20
14	Nitrite	1	0
15	Iron	1	0.3
1	Copper	1.5	0.05
17	Manganese	1	0
18	Zinc	15	5
19	Mercury	0.002	0.001
20	Lead	0.05	0.03
21	Selenium	0.01	0.005
22	Barium	0.5	0
23	Boron	5	1
24	Cadmium	0.01	0.005
25	Chromium	0.05	0.03
26	Silver	0.04	0
27	Arsenic	0.04	0.03
28	Cyanide	0.015	0
29	Phenolic compounds	0.002	0.001
30	Aluminum	0.2	0.03
31	Alkyl benzene sulfonate	0.5	0
32	Carbon chloroform extract	0.2	0
33	Chlorinated hydrocarbons	0.002	0
34	Pesticide residues	0.001	0
35	Residual free chlorine	0.3	0.2
36	Organic phosphates	0.004	0
37	Ammonia	50	0
38	Total bacterial count /ml	1	0
39	Coliform count/100 ml	10	1
40	Electrical conductivity (Reciprocal mega ohms/cm)	2500	1500

Chapter 5

Dietary Carbohydrates— Starch and Sugars

The major portion of our daily food is carbohydrates (CHO). It is made up of starch and several sugars, mainly glucose, galactose, fructose, sucrose, maltose and lactose. Starch is a polysaccharide, made up of several (α) molecules of glucose. During digestion, the starch will break down to several molecules of glucose. The structural formula of glucose and starch are shown below. They are the major source of energy for our body, followed by lipids (fats and oils) and proteins. One gram of CHO, lipids and proteins will supply 4, 9 and 4 K Calories (Kcal) of energy, respectively, to our body, after digestion and absorption. Another unusual source of energy is alcohol, which supplies 7 Kcal of energy per gram.

Structural Formula of Glucose and Starch

Besides starch and sugars, CHO consists of glycogen (also known as animal starch) and polysaccharides other than starch, which are called Non-starch Polysaccharides (NSP). This NSP is also referred to as **fiber** and is not digestible by humans. It is comprised of cellulose, hemicellulose, pectins, inulins, gums, mananoligo-saccharides, mucilages, xylans, polydextrose, beta glucans and other complex CHO. Lignin, the woody portion of plants, is not a CHO but is part of crude fiber, for all practical purposes. Cellulose, which forms a major portion of NSP, is also made up of several molecules of glucose, just like starch, but cannot be digested by humans due to lack of the enzyme cellulase in our digestive system. Herbivorous animals, especially ruminants, like cattle, can utilize cellulose for energy purpose due to the presence of microbes in their gut, which will secrete the enzyme cellulase and other NSP digesting enzymes.

Zero calorie/negative calorie foods
There are also **zero calorie** and **negative calorie foods**, which either have low calories or utilize more calories for preparation (cooking) and in eating, digestion, absorption and excretion, exceeding the calories contributed by it. Some nutritionists have classified natural foods having less than 15 calories/100 g as negative calorie foods. These foods are rich in fiber and good for weight reduction purpose. They will also satisfy hunger, due to their bulky nature, without contributing many calories.

Most of the green leafy vegetables like spinach, kale, celery and lettuce are negative calorie foods. Vegetables like okra (lady's finger), beans, broccoli, cabbage, all gourds, pumpkin, drumstick (*Moringa oleifera*), asparagus, cauliflower, cucumbers, radishes, turnips and fruits like watermelon, many berries, guava, grapefruit, lemon, apples, cranberries, oranges, papaya, pineapple, raspberries, strawberries, tangerines etc. are low calorie foods, rich in fiber.

Water has no calories. Hence, water at body temperature is a zero calorie food, whereas **cold water** is a negative calorie food, because to bring it to body temperature, some energy/calories will be utilized. However, cold water shall not be used for weight reduction purpose. Details of negative calorie foods are discussed in subsequent chapters on crude fiber and weight management.

Empty calorie foods

There is another category of foods, called **"empty calorie foods."** USDA has defined the term "empty calorie foods" as foods which supply only calories but little or no nutrients like vitamins, minerals, essential amino acids and essential fatty acids. Sugar, artificial soft drinks stuffed with sugar, hydrogenated fats, solid fats and alcohol come under this category because they supply only calories and no other nutrients. These foods are unhealthy for all, especially for diabetic and obese persons. So it is better for everyone to avoid taking these empty calories. Other nutrients/food items like vitamins, minerals, water and even cholesterol, will not supply any energy but they are have several other vital functions in our body.

Functions of CHO:

- CHO are the main source of energy (calories) to the body. Nearly 55-75 % of food energy is from CHO source only.

- Excess dietary CHO will be converted into non-essential amino acids and fatty acids. These excess fatty acids will be converted into body fat, which is unhealthy.

- Dietary fiber or NSP, even though it is not digested by humans, performs several health promoting functions in the body. Details of fiber nutrition are discussed in a separate chapter on fiber.

Why more people are becoming diabetic

Due to cholesterol phobia created in the minds of numerous people by the media, vegetarian lobby and false advisements by quacks, they are eating lots of CHO, mostly from refined and polished flour, starch and sugars at the expense of lipids and proteins, resulting in deficiency of essential amino acids, essential fatty acids, minerals and fat soluble vitamins. So typical diets in the third world countries are full of CHO and deficient in lipids and proteins. As per WHO, ADA, ICMR and other valid sources of information, low lipids and protein consumption, combined with excess CHO consumption among Indians have resulted in the world's highest and ever-growing incidences of diabetes and pre-diabetes in India.

As per the data available in 2015 from different authenticated sources like WHO, India has the fastest growing incidences of diabetes in the world. About 18.5% of the world's diabetics are in India. The actual figure must be higher than this because many millions of poor diabetic patients in rural areas are not included in this list. By the year 2020, India will have the highest number of diabetics in the world, and nearly 22% of the world's population are diabetics.

How much energy is needed and at what ratio?

The problems of elevated blood glucose level, hypercholesterolemia, diabetes and pre-diabetes can be reduced if junk food consumption is stopped. As stated earlier, a healthy man with sedentary habits needs about 2000 K. calories of energy/day, and a healthy woman with sedentary habits needs about 1,700 K.Cal./day, which is roughly equivalent to about 30 Cal./kg body weight/day. However, overweight and obese persons have to consume <25 Cal./kg/day. On the other hand, growing children, sports persons, pregnant and lactating women need >30 Cal./kg/day.

According to the dietary guidelines-RDA recommended by various countries, in a healthy adult's diet, these **daily recommended calories must be obtained from CHO, lipids and proteins, in the ideal ratio of 60:27:13** respectively, as shown in **Table-5-2.** Growing children, athletes, pregnant and lactating women need more calories from protein and lipids. Hence, for them the ratio will be 55:30:15. For diabetics also, the ideal recommended ratio will be in the range of 53-55: 28-32: 14-16, depending on other complications they have. Unfortunately, this actual ratio in India is 73; 17:10 ratio, as shown in Table-5-1, 2 and 3. This ratio is more diabeto-genic, as well as deficient in essential amino acids and fatty acids. Moreover, in India the middle and high income group consume more than the required calories, especially from refined starch, polished rice, hydrogenated fat (vanaspathi-dalda) and sugars like all bakery products, sweets, paratta, pastas, noodles, burgers and other restaurant fast foods.

CHO, especially refined flours, polished rice and sugars in the diet will be quickly digested and absorbed into the blood, compared to the lipids and proteins. Sugars will be absorbed immediately, without much digestion, shooting the blood sugar levels up. It has the highest glycemic index of 100. Hence, sugar is not advisable for diabetic patients. Junk foods are made up of sugars and refined starch which are digested and absorbed quickly, within four hours.

Table-5-1: Recommend energy (calories) contribution (%) from dietary CHO, lipids and protein in different countries

Country / Area / Organization	CHO	Lipids	Proteins
ADA & WHO's recommended ideal ratio for healthy adults	60	27	13
Ideal recommended ratio for growing children, pregnant & lactating women	55	30	15
Recommended ratio for **diabetics**	55	31	14
World average ratio	64	25	11
Developed countries ratio	54	34	12
Developing countries ratio	67	22	11
Asia	67	22	11
Africa	73	18	9
Latin America	63	26	11
USA	49	39	12
INDIA	**73**	**17**	**10**
UK	52	36	12
France	46	41	13
Germany	51	37	12
Spain	46	41	13
Italy	49	39	12
Japan	59	28	13

- Among the countries cited above, Japanese people are consuming energy from different sources, close to the recommended levels.

- Developed countries, especially Europeans are consuming more than the recommended energy from lipids and less from CHO. Hence, the incidence of diabetes is low in Europe and high in Asia.

- On the other hand, **Indians are getting the highest energy from CHO (see also table-5-2),** higher than poor Afro-Asian countries. Since CHO have high glycemic index, Indians have the highest incidence of diabetes in the world. This also leads to more heart diseases, as observed by Dr. Dwight Lundell (2015), which will be discussed in detail in other chapters.

- Average **Indian diets are deficient in both proteins and lipids and excess in CHO. Hence, our recommendations to our people are to consume lesser quantities of refined starchy and sugary foods and increase the consumptions of healthy oils and proteins.**

Excess blood glucose will be converted into body fat, especially as highly saturated stearic acid, because the body cannot synthesize essential unsaturated fatty acids. Excess blood glucose, which cannot be absorbed into the tissues, also will irritate the arterial walls, just like trans-fatty acids and free radicals, which act as abrasive materials and damage the arterial walls, over which the cholesterol will be deposited as flakes, blocking the free flow of blood in the arteries and capillaries, resulting in CVD and stroke.

Table-5-2: NIN Recommended Dietary Allowances (RDA) for Indians

Sex & extent of physical activity: man's average body weight = 65 kg & woman's = 55 kg	NIN RDA-Energy= calories /day	Protein = g	Visible + invisible lipids /day-g	% Calories supplied by:		
				CHO	Lipids	Proteins
Man: Sedentary work	2320	60	25 +10 =35	76.1	13.6	10.3
Man: Moderate work	2730	60	30+10 =40	78.0	13.2	8.80
Man: Active work	3490	60	40 +10 =50	80.2	12.9	6.90
Woman: Sedentary work	1900	55	20 +10 =30	74.2	14.2	11.6
Woman: Moderate work	2230	55	25 +10 = 35	76.04	14.1	9.86
Woman: Active work	2850	55	30 +10 =40	79.68	12.6	7.72

Table-5-3: USDA/ ADA/ Chinese /Japanese /Europe's FNB recommended energy levels

Sex & extent of physical activity (man's average body weight = 70 kg & woman's = 60 kg)	Energy = calories /day	Protein = g	Total lipids /day-g	% Calories supplied by:		
				CHO	Lipids	Proteins
Man: Sedentary work	2200	70	70	58.7	28.6(29)	12.7
Man: Moderate work	2400	70	75	59.4	28.1(28)	12.5
Man: Active work	2600	75	80	60.0	27.7(28)	12.3
Woman: Sedentary work	1600	55	53	56.5	29.8(30)	13.7
Woman: Moderate work	1800	60	60	56.7	30	13.3
Woman: Active work	2000	65	66	57.3	29.7(30)	13.0

Even though NIN has recommended 20-30% calories of lipid origin in its manual in one place, the total visible + invisible lipids recommended in its RDA in the same manual supplies <15 % calories only, resulting in more calories of CHO origin. These excess calories recommended by NIN, as shown in Table 5-2, especially more calories of CHO origin and less calories of lipid and protein origin, are contrary to the recommendations of many other countries and several scientists, as shown in **Table-5-3.** These types of outdated and confusing recommendations have resulted in more incidences of diabetes, obesity, hyper-cholesterol, hypertension, CVD, arthritis, osteoporosis and cancer in India. Dr. Mark Hyman (2016) is recommending, **"Eat Fat & Get Thin"**, without increasing the total calorie intake, for weight reduction.

How to calculate your daily energy requirements
The American Dietetic Association has given "**Mifflin-St Jeor**" formulas for calculating the daily energy requirements. First, we have to calculate the Basal Energy Requirement (BER) as follows:

Men= 10 x weight in kg + 6.25 x height in cm - 5 x age in years + 5

Women= 10 x weight in kg + 6.25 x height in cm - 5 x age in years – 161

These calories are the basic calories needed for a bed-ridden person, with zero physical activity i.e. BER. But every person will have some level of physical activity. So, to arrive at the actual calories needed, we have to multiply this BER with the **body activity factor**; which ranges from 1.2 to 1.9, depending on their physical activity.

- 1.2 to 1.4= for persons with low physical activity or sedentary habits
- 1.5 to 1.6= for persons with moderate physical activity
- 1.7 to 1.8= for persons with high physical activity
- 1.9 = for sports persons

According to this formula, a 60-year-old man, weighing 70 kg, with 170 cm height and sedentary habits, the BER will be;

- (10X70 + 6.25X 170) – (5X60) +5= 700+1062.5 or say 1063=1763 - 300+5=1458 X1.2 (sedentary) =1750 calories /day.

If the person is a woman, with the same data, then her daily calories requirements will be,

- 1763- 300-161= 1302 X 1.2= 1562 calories / day

This provides us the maintenance calories required/day. If we consume these calories daily, there will not be any weight gain or loss. If you want to lose body weight, 10 -20% lesser calories may be consumed. Moreover, this calorie restriction must be gradual. Never go beyond 40 % calorie restriction or a maximum of 500 calories cut per day. Restrict mainly CHO calories as far as possible and never cut protein calories, unless you have some kidney problem or under medical advice.

Excess calorie consumption beyond the requirements of the body, irrespective of the source, will be converted to **glycogen**, also called animal starch, to a limited extent and stored in muscles and liver, which may be sufficient for a day. However, the major portion of excess dietary energy, whatever may be its source (CHO, Lipids or Proteins) will be converted into body fat, especially as saturated fat, since the human body cannot synthetize essential unsaturated fatty acids like PUFA. This will result in overweight and obesity. On the other hand, lower calories consumption will utilize glycogen, stored in the liver and muscles initially for energy, followed by depletion of body fat and ultimately body protein as body fuel, resulting in weight loss, general weakness and low disease resistance capacity.

Lipids and proteins take longer for digestion and absorption, ranging from 6 to 12 hours, depending on the nature of foods consumed, cooking method and the individuals' ability for digestion. Hence, they have low glycemic index. Presence of fiber in the food also slows down digestion and absorption of nutrients. Fiber also binds with cholesterol in the diet as well as in the bile, through which the internal cholesterol will be expelled into the intestine and the fiber-bound cholesterol will come out through stools from the body. If a person consumes slightly excess lipids and protein, but the total calories consumed are within the stipulated levels, i.e. low CHO-normal calorie diet, there won't be any harm to the body because this excess lipid and proteins will be utilized for energy purpose and not deposited as body fat.

Dr. Dwight Lundell, (2015), a leading cardiac surgeon, Dr. Bereliami (2016), a leading cardiologist, and many other eminent physicians (Drs. Marl Merrill, Meridan Zenner, Mark Hyman, Oz, Robert etc.) have concluded that excess blood glucose, oxidized trans-fatty acids (present in hydrogenated fats like vanaspathi, margarines, over-boiled oils during continuous deep frying) and other free radicals (oxidative materials) will cause constant irritation and inflammation to the blood vessel walls and damage them. Over the damaged blood vessel walls, the LDL cholesterol and other waxy materials will be deposited and block/narrow the blood vessels. Without this inflammation and damage to the arterial walls, there is no way that cholesterol will deposit over the walls of the blood vessels, causing CVD and strokes. Without inflammation, the cholesterol will move freely throughout the body as nature intended. It is the inflammation that causes cholesterol to become trapped. Hence, **cholesterol is not the culprit for CVD; the culprits are the inflammatory materials mentioned above.**

Dr. Roy Taylor (2016) of New Castle University, UK, has concluded that fat deposits around the pancreas and fatty infiltration are the prime causes for its inability to secrete enough insulin. When we consume more processed carbohydrates, such as sugar and starch (replacing fats) having high glycemic index, the blood sugar rises rapidly. In response, the pancreas secretes insulin, which drives the sugar into each cell, where it is stored for energy. If insulin is deficient, the glucose storage capacity of the cells decreases and the cells will reject the extra glucose. These extra sugar molecules attach to a variety of proteins, called as "**apo-proteins**", which will act as an abrasive material and injure the walls of the blood vessels over which the cholesterol will be deposited. This extra blood glucose will be converted into body fat, leading to obesity, high blood pressure, diabetes, dementia, stroke, Alzheimer's disease etc. Moreover, the overloaded fat cells (adipose tissue) pour out large quantities of pro-inflammatory chemicals, like free radicals, which further damage the arterial walls.

Millets are more healthy grains
Millets are minor grains, also called ancient grains, grown in small quantities in tropical countries, mainly as rain fed crops. Their yields and availability are lesser compared to major grains like wheat, rice, corn, oats and barley. However, their nutritional values are far superior to the major grains, due to their high fiber, complex CHO, lower glycemic index, lower energy and higher micronutrients availability. Besides supplying fiber and micronutrients, they have special health promoting functions, like control of Asthma, I.B.S., diabetes and other conditions, as shown in **Table- 5-4**.

Table-5-4: Common millets and their functions

Scientific name	Common names	Special health promoting functions
Echinochloa spp.	Barn yard millet, Japanese barnyard millet, kudhiraival, kodisama, udalu, burgu millet	Liver tonic, prevents gall stones
Eleusine coracana	Finger millet, ragi, kezhvaragu	Controls diabetes, IBS, asthma
Pennisetum glaucum	Pearl millet, cambu, bajra, *Sajjalu*	Increases breast milk, corrects irregular menses cycle
Panicum miliaceum	Proso millet, broom corn millet, hog millet, white millet, Pani-varagu	Detoxification of the body
Panicum sumatrense	Little millet samai, samalu	Corrects menstrual disorders
Paspalum scrobiculatum	Kodo millet, varagu, arikalu, koden	Blood purifier
Setaria italica	Fox tail millet, thenai, korralu	Prevents nervous debilities, proper fetus growth
Sorghum vulgare	*Milo, jonna,* cholam Jowar	Prevents IBS
Urochloa spp.	Brown top millet, Brachiaria, Guinea millet	Controls diabetes, IBS

Other ancient minor millets are spelt, freekeh, quinoa, teff, chia, farro, amaranth, kamut etc. These millets can substitute major grains for better health, weight management and are especially suitable for diabetes patients and pre-diabetics to reduce cholesterol, blood pressure and other chronic diseases. They can be consumed through multi-grain breads, soups, porridge, gruel, upma, pongal and other local dishes at least once a day or 3 to 4 times a week, substituting major grains, especially replacing unhealthy refined flour and polished rice.

Many health authorities in India are still recommending higher energy levels of 2400-2800 K.Cal./day for Indians, that too from CHO, resulting in obesity. On the other hand, many countries are recommending lower energy levels ranging from 1600 to 2000 K.Cal./day for their people, equivalent to 28 Cal./kg body weight/day, depending on gender and physical activity. In general, men and women with sedentary habits need less than 2000 and 1700 K.Cal. of energy/day, respectively. This energy will be supplied by CHO, lipids and proteins, in the ratios mentioned in Table-5-1. Excess energy from any of these sources will be converted into body saturated fat, resulting in increase in the body weight. However, if the total energy is deficient, the body fat will be utilized for energy purpose, resulting in body weight loss. If a person consumes more saturated fats, but the total energy consumed is within the limits (<2000 /1700 Kcal.), then this entire saturated fat, as well as some body fat, will be burnt for energy purpose. In such case, where is the question of dietary saturated fat causing the harm to the health, if the total calorie consumed is within the limits?

If a person consumes well-balanced food, but with excess total daily energy requirement from any source, it will be converted into body fat. **Therefore, the real problem here is the excess calorie intake, especially from CHO origin and not the saturated fat (SFA). In fact, of late the ADA, AHA and USDA are recommending up to 20 g of dietary SFA alone, which contributes about 10% of total dietary calories; whereas, the Indian authorities are recommending very low fat and high CHO diet, resulting in diabetes.**

How much CHO, lipids and proteins do we need daily?
As stated above, a healthy man with a sedentary lifestyle needs about 2000 Kcal. of energy per day. In a healthy diet, these 2000 calories must be derived from CHO, lipids and proteins, in the ratio of 60:27:13. This is equivalent to 1200 + 540 + 260 calories of energy from CHO, lipids and proteins, respectively. At the rate of 4, 9 and 4 Kcal. of energy/g of CHO, lipids and proteins, respectively, a person needs 300 g of CHO, 60 g of lipids and 65 g of proteins (about 1 g protein/kg body weight/day) daily. Assuming that a person will get 2% invisible/bound fat/residual oil from cereals, pulses, vegetables and fruits to the tune of 500 g, he will get about 10 g of

lipids from invisible sources. The remaining 50 g (60-10=50 g or 55 ml) must be supplemental (added) lipids. However, the actual per capita oil consumption in many developing countries at present is as low as 30 ml of added oil/day, with proportionate increase in the CHO content, resulting in the world's highest incidence of diabetes in India.

Fundamentals of biochemistry say that CHO, lipids and proteins are interconvertible in the body, with the exception of essential fatty acids and amino acids. If the total calories exceed the limits prescribed for the individuals, the excess calories, whatever may be the origin, will be converted into body saturated fat, mainly stearic acid, resulting in obesity. **Hence, avoid excess consumption of calories, especially of CHO origin, especially from refined CHO and sugar, to prevent diabetes, CVD and obesity.**

Chapter 6

Dietary Fiber

Fiber is the indigestible portion of our foods of plant origin that passes through our digestive tract. Fiber is indigestible in humans, but herbivorous animals and ruminants can digest it better, by the microorganisms present in their digestive tract. Fiber is not a nutrient, not digested and absorbed in humans, but it performs several health promoting functions within the food and digestive tract. Except lignin (woody portion), all other fiber materials are complex carbohydrate, which includes cellulose, hemicellulose, pectins, pentosans, inulins, gums, manan-oligosaccharides, glucan-oligosaccharides, mucilages, xylans, polydextrins, beta-glucans and other complex CHO. They are also called Non-Starch Polysaccharides (NSP). Cellulose forms the major portion of the fiber/NSP.

A few decades back, people were consuming unpolished whole grains, like brown rice, wheat, barley, oats, rye, triticale, various millets (also called ancient grains—some of them are, amaranth, bran millet, chia, farro, finger millet, foxtail millet, freekeh, kamut, pearl millet, quinoa, teff etc.), milo (Jowar), maize (corn), barley, beans, peas, lentils, pulses, nuts etc. as whole unrefined and unpolished products, rich in bran (fiber). This fiber will bind with cholesterol (both dietary and endogenous in bile) and prevent its absorption by excretion in the stool. Fiber also makes foods bulkier, helps in excretion of waste in stools, and prevents constipation, diverticulitis and colon cancer. Moreover, these brans, fiber and complex carbo-hydrates in the whole grains, beans, peas and nuts, takes more time for digestion and absorption. Hence, they have lower glycemic index compared to junk foods having refined flour, polished grains and sugars that we are consuming at present.

All fiber rich foods have few calories and are considered **"negative calorie foods"** because the energy spent by the body to prepare, cook, eat and digest them is higher than the energy supplied by them. So we will be losing energy during their digestion and absorption. Diets having more fiber are bulky, require more chewing time, take longer time for digestion and maintain healthy peristaltic movement of the intestine.

Fiber requirements:
Growing children need 15 to 25 grams of fiber per day for good health, depending on their age. Women and men need 25 and 38 g/day, respectively. These requirements decrease after 50 years of age. These levels can be met by consuming whole grains rich in bran, about 100 to 200 g of mixed fruits and vegetables and 50 to 100 g of green leafy vegetables daily. Diabetic and obese persons can consume up to 50 g fiber/day to control blood sugar levels and reduce body weight. However, in developed countries, people are getting only about 15 grams a day, resulting in constipation, diverticulitis and colon cancer. On the other hand, people in poor Afro-Asian countries consume more than 50 g fiber per day, which affects the digestion and absorption of nutrients. Therefore, both low and high fiber diets are not good for health. Hence, Narahari et al.(1993) recommended 25 -40 g of fiber/day or 1 to 2 % for every 1000 calorie energy consumption or 1% of daily food intake, with equal proportions of soluble and insoluble fibers.

In humans, the fiber passes through the digestive tract, so it is less likely to cause blood sugar to spike. In fact, individuals with diabetes who ate 50 grams of fiber a day had better blood sugar control than those who ate considerably less. High fiber foods are also recommended for obese persons for body weight control. Consume daily 50-100 g of negative calorie foods like green leafy vegetables, and high fiber- low-calorie- non/low- sweet fruits like various berries, pineapple, wood apple, guava, kiwi and other locally available fresh fruits.

The fiber in wheat bran, oat bran, psyllium husk and whole millets is considered more effective than fiber from fruits and vegetables. Experts recommend increasing fiber intake gradually rather than suddenly, and because fiber absorbs water, beverage intake should be increased as fiber intake increases.

Source of fiber:
All green leafy vegetables; unpolished whole grains, especially millets, oats, barley, quinoa; whole beans, legumes, peas; husks/brans, especially psyllium husk; and most of the vegetables and fruits are rich sources of fiber. Polishing and refining of grains and beans will remove the outer fiber portion, which is not a recommended procedure.

Types of fiber:
There are two main types of dietary fiber: **soluble and insoluble**. Both are beneficial for health if present in foods at recommended levels.

- Soluble fiber dissolves in water. It is present in millets, oats, nuts, beans, lentils, apples, mangoes, berries and many other fruits. It holds water, turns into a gel in the intestine, adds bulk to the stool and thereby relieves constipation, flatulence and other tummy troubles. It also helps to lower both blood glucose and blood cholesterol levels.

- Insoluble fiber will not dissolve in water. It promotes peristaltic movement of the gut and thereby helps the food to move through the digestive system, promotes regularity and prevents constipation. Foods rich in insoluble fiber include whole wheat, whole wheat bread, whole grain couscous, brown rice, legumes, carrots, cucumbers, tomatoes, coconut and many leafy vegetables. Fiber also helps to lower serum cholesterol levels. A landmark study at Boston's Harvard University showed that men who consumed the highest levels of dietary fiber (around 1% of diet) had a 40% lower risk of heart disease. The main sources of fiber in this study were vegetables, fruits and whole cereals.

Excess dietary fiber:

On the other hand, eating more high fiber foods having more than 50 g of dietary fiber per day (>1% of the diet) causes indigestion and stomach upset. Fiber also binds with other nutrients like minerals and vitamins in the diet, reducing their absorption and increasing their elimination. Hence, we have to limit its availability in our foods to the recommended levels only. However, diabetic and obese persons can go for slightly higher fiber diets in order to control blood sugar level and body weight, respectively. In such case, they must take vitamin and mineral supplementation to meet losses.

Some tips for increasing fiber intake:

- Consume whole unpolished grains, beans and nuts.
- Do not peel the outer skin of many fruits and vegetables. Use them as whole, unless their skin/shell is very tough.
- Eat whole fruits instead of drinking fruit juices and sodas.
- Replace white rice, bread, and pasta with brown rice and whole grain products.
- Snack on raw vegetables and fruits instead of chips, crackers, chocolate bars or any junk foods.
- Consume boiled whole beans or legumes with skin.
- Eat sprouted grains and lentils (pulses) as salads.
- Eat salads without any sauce or dips having sugar or high energy.
- Replace part of rice, corn and wheat with whole millets and oats.
- Consume at least 100 g of fresh mixed green leaves daily, preferably as salads.
-

Table-6-1: How dietary fiber works?

Fiber In the:	Fiber actions	Fiber benefits to our health
Stomach and small intestine	• causes a sense of fullness • traps cholesterol and fats • slows absorption of sugars	• regulates weight • binds & eliminates cholesterol • controls blood glucose level
Large intestine	• causes fermentation, promotes growth of healthy probiotic bacteria • absorbs water, adding "bulk" to stool • prevents diverticulitis, colo-rectal cancer and piles	• enhances the immune system to fight infection and chronic diseases • promotes peristaltic movement of intestine & prevents constipation • Promotes probiosis. Fiber & probiotic microorganisms have symbiotic effect.

Functions of fiber:

- Diets having more fiber require more chewing time, so it takes a longer time to eat and digest the food. Your body recognizes this and feels full sooner, resulting in lesser calorie intake and body weight control. This is why increasing the dietary fiber intake will aid in **weight loss and weight maintenance** efforts. In particular, fiber may reduce abdominal obesity, which is part of a cluster of symptoms known as metabolic syndrome that increase the risk of heart disease.

- Fiber makes the food bulky, helps to maintain healthy peristaltic movement of the digestive track and thereby prevents constipation, diverticulitis and colon cancer.

- Fiber binds and excretes cholesterol (both dietary and endogenous from bile) and thereby reduces serum cholesterol levels.

- A large-scale study during 2016 led by researchers at Harvard T. H. Chan School of Public Health showed that women who ate more high-fiber foods during adolescence and young adulthood, including vegetables and fruit, may have significantly lower breast cancer risk than those who eat less dietary fiber when young.

- Diverticulitis, an inflammation of the intestine, is one of the most common age-related disorders of the colon in Western society. Among male health professionals in a long-term follow-up study, eating dietary fiber, particularly insoluble fiber, was associated with about a 40 percent lower risk of diverticular disease.

- Diets low in fiber and high in foods that cause sudden increases in blood sugar may increase the risk of developing type 2 diabetes. Both Harvard studies—of female nurses and of male health professionals—found that this type of diet more than doubled the risk of type 2 diabetes when compared to a diet high in cereal fiber and low in high-glycemic-index foods. A diet high in cereal fiber was linked to a lower risk of type 2 diabetes

- In fact, individuals with diabetes who ate 50 grams of fiber a day had better blood sugar control than those who ate considerably less. Consume daily 50-100 g of negative calorie foods like green leafy vegetables, high fiber- low-calorie- non-/low- sweet fruits like various berries, wood apple, guava and other locally available fresh seasonal fruits.

- Soluble fiber controls hemorrhoids and diverticulitis (inflammation of the intestine), as well as relieving some of the symptoms of irritable bowel syndrome (IBS), such as diarrhea, abdominal pain and gas.

- Insoluble fiber binds with dietary (exogenous) and bile cholesterol (endogenous) and eliminates them from the body through stools. As such, the fiber helps in eliminating excess cholesterol from the body and food. A landmark study at Boston's Harvard University showed that men who consumed the highest levels of dietary fiber (>1% of diet) had a 40% lower risk of heart disease. The main sources of fiber in this study were vegetables, fruits and whole cereal.

- Fiber helps to regulate the body's use of sugars, helping to keep hunger and blood sugar in check. Fiber helps in weight management, lowering the glycemic index and maintaining satiety. Eating more fiber-rich vegetables, fruits and beans can reduce belly fat. For every 10-gram increase in fiber eaten per day, belly fat will be reduced by almost 4% within a year.

- Fiber helps in maintaining normal gut micro-flora and thereby promotes probiosis.

- High intake of dietary fiber has been linked to a lower risk of heart disease in a number of large studies that followed people for many years. In a Harvard study of over 40,000 male health professionals and female nurses, researchers found that a high total dietary fiber intake was linked to a 40 percent lower risk of coronary heart disease.

Higher fiber intake has also been linked to a lower risk of metabolic syndrome, a combination of factors that increases the risk of developing heart disease and diabetes. These factors include high blood pressure, low insulin levels, excess weight (especially around the abdomen), high levels of triglycerides and low levels of HDL (good) cholesterol. Several studies suggest that higher intake of fiber may offer protective benefits from this syndrome. High fiber diets also prevent colon cancer, constipation and piles.

Chapter 7

Cholesterol Myths and Facts

The common public is scared of cholesterol and many times are misguided by a few health care professionals who have not updated their technical skills. Science has now proved beyond doubt that serum cholesterol is independent of dietary cholesterol, and that many other factors are responsible for cholesterol deposition in the arteries, blocking free flow of blood and causing CVD. The details are discussed in this chapter.

Cholesterol is classified under lipids, because it is soluble in fat solvents like hexane and ethanol. It is a soft, waxy substance found in animal fats and oils. Unlike CHO, fats, oils and proteins, cholesterol will not supply any calories/energy to the body. It is not dietary essential, because our body can synthesize as much cholesterol as it requires. However, **cholesterol is essential to the body, because it is the structural component of nervous tissue, cell membrane, endocrine glands, liver and other tissues which perform many vital functions in the body. Humans and other animals cannot survive in the absence of cholesterol, because it is the mother (base material) of many hormones and several biochemical substances in the body, like bile and vitamin D.**

How much cholesterol our body can synthesize?
One cannot avoid or reduce serum cholesterol simply by avoiding dietary cholesterol, because our body can synthesize as much as 2000 mg of cholesterol per day of which nearly 80%

is by liver and the remaining cholesterol synthesis will be in intestine, skin, kidneys, adrenal cortex, aorta, spleen and muscles. So there is no RDA for it, but it is an essential component of the body. **It is not at all a harmful substance. It is a normal constituent of the human body. About 0.2% of a healthy adult body weight is cholesterol.** Hence, a person weighing 70 kg, contains about 140 g of cholesterol in the body, mostly in the brain and other nervous tissues. It is also found in large amounts in the liver, kidney and in the blood stream.

Cholesterol structural formula:

Cholesterol scare:

Many people in the world, especially those above 40 years of age, are much afraid of cholesterol—called **"Cholesterol Scare"**—without understanding much about it. Added to this, many ill-informed professional persons, without updating their technical knowledge on cholesterol and nutrition, are conveying outdated information on cholesterol to the public and causing them to be afraid of cholesterol. **Meta-analysis of epidemiological data and latest research from many universities has proven beyond doubt that dietary cholesterol has little role in elevating serum cholesterol, and that these two are independent entities.** Since the body can synthesize enough cholesterol, raised serum cholesterol is not due to dietary cholesterol but is due to failure in the body mechanism to eliminate excess serum cholesterol, due to various factors, which are discussed in this chapter. **Based on reliable evidences, in 2014 the ADA and AHA have removed the cholesterol intake limit of 300 mg/day.**

To get rid of this cholesterol scare, people need to thoroughly understand cholesterol's role in the human body and metabolism. At the same time, people must be more careful with the real culprits: the junk foods and processed foods like artificial aerated soft drinks, many bakery products, cookies, French fries, chips, sweets, and many processed and further processed foods, which are more health hazardous because they contain **various harmful food additives/chemicals, sugar, refined flour (maida/all-purpose flour), hydrogenated fats (vanaspathi), trans-fatty acids, free radicals etc.** In spite of repeated advice from health authorities to not consume junk foods and processed foods, many people are still attracted to them and spoil their health by continuing to consume them.

Cholesterol requirements and biosynthesis:
The average daily requirement of cholesterol for an adult is about 1200 mg. This can be either supplemented in the diet or entirely synthesized in the body, mostly by the latter. The average daily consumption of cholesterol in developed countries is about 300 mg/day; whereas in the developing countries it is less than 140 mg, and in India as well as in some poor Afro-Asian countries, it is less than 60 mg/day. Moreover, the dietary cholesterol absorption rate varies from 15 to 71 % (average 40%) and is inversely proportional to the level of cholesterol in the food. So only about 40% of dietary cholesterol is absorbed. Hence, the body will synthesize the remaining daily requirements of cholesterol, mainly in the liver and the intestine. Dietary plant sterols (phytostrols) like sitosterol present in vegetables, fruits and nuts, cholestyramine, fiber, neomycin, nicotinic acid (but not nicotinamide) will decrease the cholesterol biosynthesis and/or absorption from intestine. Nearly 80 % of cholesterol will be converted into **cholic acid**.

Even vegans, who consume '0'mg of cholesterol, will have enough cholesterol in the body, due to biosynthesis. So vegans and vegetarians are also not exempted from hypercholesterolemia. Our body can synthesize enough cholesterol (endogenous), from simple 2-carbon fragments like acetates and acetyl Co-A, for which the enzyme, "Hydroxy Methyl Glutaryl Coenzyme-A Reductase" acts as a catalyst. McCharen (1989) stated that in healthy persons, the sum of endogenous (synthesized) and exogenous (dietary) cholesterol, for a given period, is more or less constant. **Therefore, to reduce the serum cholesterol, dietary cholesterol reduction is not the answer. We have to find out the real reasons, like processed-junk foods consumption, excess calorie intake, lack of exercise etc.**

If cholesterol is available in the food, its biosynthesis will be proportionately reduced by feedback mechanism. **A healthy vegan, who consumes '0' mg cholesterol, will have normal serum cholesterol levels due to sufficient cholesterol biosynthesis. On the other hand, Eskimos, who consume the highest (>2000 mg/day) dietary cholesterol per day, will have normal serum cholesterol levels, due to low biosynthesis or quick excretion of it. These findings have clearly indicated that there is no co-relationship between dietary cholesterol and serum cholesterol.** American Dietetic Association and many authorities also arrived at similar conclusions.

Furthermore, extensive research work carried out by W.H.O., F.A.O., many universities, Multiple Risk Factor Intervention Trail Research groups of (M.R.F.I.T.), Committee on Medical Aspects of Food Policy (C.O.M.A.), American Heart Association (A.H.A.), American Dietetic Association (A.D.A.), Department of Health and Social Security of U.K., National Cholesterol Education Program of the Heart, Lung and Blood Institute (N.C.E.P.H.L.B.I.) of U.S.A. etc. revealed that serum cholesterol level is independent of dietary cholesterol level and that these two are independent entities. In a joint study conducted at three locations (Atlanta, Minneapolis & New Orleans, USA), involving 3000 volunteers consuming 1 to 21 eggs per week (30 to 621 mg of cholesterol /day), noticed no significant variations in the serum cholesterol levels, based on their cholesterol consumption.

Based on these reliable findings, the American Dietetic Association (ADA) has lifted the upper ceiling of 300 mg cholesterol per day in 2014 and now there is no restriction on cholesterol consumption in their RDA values. Many other countries also, have not prescribed any upper limit for cholesterol consumption, but still NIN of India is advising to restrict the cholesterol intake to less than 200 mg/day, based on the outdated information. In fact, the average dietary cholesterol consumption in India is a meagre 60 mg/day, which is one of the lowest in the world. Then what is the necessity for further reduction of cholesterol intake, and how it is going to improve the health of the individuals?

Why should we consume cholesterol?
A question arises, why should we consume cholesterol when there is no dietary requirement (RDA) for it, due to biosynthesis? The answer is that if you want to eliminate cholesterol consumption totally, you should not consume any animal products, including milk, eggs and fish, which are rich in high biological value protein, all vitamins, minerals, anti-diabetic tasty foods having low glycemic index, giving good satiety and several other health benefits. Moreover, many essential nutrients like vitamin-B12, D3, carnosine, creatine, EPA, DHA, taurine and many essential amino acids are abundant in foods of animal origin, which are either deficient or absent in foods of plant origin. Foods of animal origin are good for diabetic patients because they are low glycemic index foods. Since our body can synthesize enough cholesterol, "0-cholesterol foods" are of no use to reduce serum cholesterol. At the same time, they are depriving of valuable nutrients from foods of animal origin. Hence, for obtaining valuable essential nutrients from animal foods and as part of a balanced healthy diet, there is no harm in consuming cholesterol, along with nutritious animal foods; otherwise, there will be more cholesterol biosynthesis.

Cholesterol functions in our body:

- Cholesterol is the base material for synthesis of most of the hormones, enzymes, bile, Vitamin-D, and is the **mother of all hormones.**
- It is the essential component of all nervous tissues and performs many vital metabolic functions in the body, like neuron-transmission. Without cholesterol, there is no brain and nervous tissue.
- Cholesterol is required for digestion. As a constituent of bile, it helps in fat emulsification and digestion.
- As a constituent of various hormones and enzymes, it performs innumerable life-saving metabolic functions in the body.
- As a constituent of male and female reproductive hormones, testosterone, estrogen etc. it controls all reproductive activities like semen production, menstrual cycle, egg/ovum production, fetus growth and child birth.
- Unlike other lipids, CHO and proteins, cholesterol does not supply any energy to the body.
- As a normal constituent of cell membrane, cholesterol is essential for new tissues formation; which will replace old /dead tissues.
- Cholesterol will protect and insulate nerve fibers and nervous tissue.
- It aids in the transportation and metabolism of fatty acids, triglycerides and fat-soluble vitamins in the body.
- Cholesterol maintains the structure of chylomicrons which is an essential component of lipoproteins.
- Cholesterol neutralizes certain natural toxins like saponins and other toxic metabolites.
- Cholesterol is a normal constituent of sebum, secreted by the sebaceous glands of the skin.

- **Hence, there is no animal kingdom without cholesterol.** AHA, MRFIT, NCCAAHA, NCEP, NCEPHLBI and resent surveys in many developed countries where the birth rate is low, as well as in several animal studies, where the fertility rate is low, gave evidence that these abnormalities are linked to low serum cholesterol and reproductive hormone levels.

Causes of elevated serum cholesterols:

As mentioned in other places in this book, as well as in this author's earlier books on, *Cholesterol-myths and facts* and *Cholesterol, fats and healthy diet*, nearly 70 % of the reasons for elevated serum cholesterol are non-dietary causes, and only 30 % are due to dietary causes, as shown in **Table-7-1**. Even among these 30 % dietary causes for raised serum cholesterol levels, dietary cholesterol is not directly or indirectly responsible for it. Excess calorie intake, consumption of refined CHO rich foods, junk foods, lack of dietary fiber and unhealthy food habits, as mentioned in Table-7-1, are responsible for elevated serum cholesterol levels. Probably, low fiber foods, high calorie intake and the chemicals (food additives) in the junk foods, may trigger the body to produce more cholesterol or prevents its excretion, as a body's defense mechanism.

Makinen and Rajakangas (1988) of the department of Nutrition, University of Helsinki, Finland, after a prolonged study involving 400 healthy volunteers, have concluded that consumption of two eggs/day, having 400 mg cholesterol /day, did not show any significant change in the serum cholesterol levels in 86% of volunteers (non-responders); 11 % are moderate responders and only 3% showed significant response for dietary cholesterol levels, which may be due to their genetic nature. Such individuals can be easily identified and take low cholesterol foods, containing not more than 200 mg/day. Hence, these guidelines have to be taken into account to reduce serum total cholesterol and LDLC.

Table-7-1: Causes of elevated serum cholesterol – Narahari *et al.* (1984)

Non-dietary causes for elevated serum cholesterols	Extent they are responsible (Approx. %)
Heredity (genetic causes- racial background, family history)	20%
Obesity/overweight- >25 BMI & hormonal imbalance	15%
Sedentary habits- lack of or insufficient physical work	10%
Other metabolic diseases like diabetes, liver and kidney disorders, hypothyroidism and metabolic dysfunctions (in women during pregnancy & breast feeding, which are healthy & temporary)	10%
Emotional stress, tension, depression, worries spoiled family relationships/friendships and other psychological problems, old age	8%
Chain smoking, chronic alcoholism, drug misuse	7%
TOTAL OF NON-DIETARY CAUSES:	**70%**
DIETARY CAUSES:	**30%**
Consumption of processed & junk foods rich in sugars, hydrogenated fats, trans-fatty acids and food additives (various chemicals) having free radicals	9%
Excess calorie consumption, especially of sugar & refined CHO origin, overeating	7%
Lack of fiber/insufficient fiber in the diet, few vegetables, greens and fruits	5%
Unhealthy food habits, like fasting & feasting, taking 1 or heavy meals instead of 4-6 split meals, untimely food intake, sleeping or doing heavy work soon after eating et	5%
Imbalanced diets, improper distribution of calories from CHO, lipids and proteins and with-in lipids	4%
TOTAL DIETARY CAUSES:	**30%**

Elevated serum cholesterol is a complex physiological / pathological phenomenon, controlled by several factors. The major dietary factors responsible for elevated serum cholesterol and triglycerides are excess dietary energy intake, eating junk foods and imbalanced foods rich in trans-fatty acids, refined CHO, sugars and free radicals. Excess calories and CHO will be converted into body fat, resulting in obesity. Among non-dietary causes, heredity, lack of exercise i.e. sedentary habits and lifestyle, tension, emotional stress (not physical stress), smoking etc., as described in Table-7-1 are responsible for elevated serum cholesterol levels.

Diet vs. serum cholesterol levels:
Dietary cholesterol and serum cholesterol are two different entities. Dietary cholesterol is found only in animal fats and oils. It is not found in any vegetable oils and fats. There is no bad or good cholesterol of food origin. Only based on its linkage with **"lipoproteins"** during transportation in the body, it is classified as HDL (High Density Lipoproteins), LDL (Low Density Lipoproteins) and VLDL (Very Low Density Lipoproteins) cholesterols. High level of HDLC (exceeding 50 mg/dl), or what doctors call good cholesterol, helps to excrete cholesterol from the body and thereby prevents damage to the arteries and heart attacks. As shown in **Table-7-2**, Europeans, especially Mediterranean, usually will have >55 mg/dl HDLC and have lesser incidence of CVD. On the other hand, American blacks and Afro-Asians will have higher incidence of CVD due to low HDLC **(<45 mg/dl). If the serum HDLC is below 40 mg/dl, the chance of suffering from a coronary artery** disease (CAD) is rather high. In general, a high serum HDLC level is an indication of prompt excretion of excess body cholesterol. Conversely, high serum LDLC and VLDLC levels are indications of poor excretion of body cholesterol and its accumulation in the body.

Table-7-2: Effect of serum cholesterol levels on CVD risk

Gender	At CVD risk	Desirable	Remarks
Men	HDLC<40 mg/dl (<1.03 mmol/L)	HDLC >55 mg/dl (>1.43 mmol/L)	Genetically, such high levels of HDLC is not noticed in Indians and Africans, for whom 45 mg/dl and above is desirable.

Women	HDLC < 45 mg/dl (<1.16 mmol/L)	HDLC >60 mg/dl (>1.55 mmol/L) or above	---do---
Men	LDLC >150mg /dl (3.89mmol/L)	LDLC <125mg/dl (3.23mmol/ L)	High CHO + high calorie diet + junk foods having trans-fatty acids + free radicals + sedentary lifestyle, increases serum LDLC
Women	LDLC>155 mg/dl (4.09mmol/L)	LDLC <130mg/dl (3.36mmol/ L)	---do---

Kay and Trusswell (1977), Mahley et al (1978), Bowden et al. (1984), Nagarajan and Narahari (2001) and Kripakaran and Narahari (2004) did not notice any significant increase in serum cholesterol levels between individuals consuming 200 to 630 mg/day. Similarly, MRFIT conducted the most extensive study involving 12,866 men aged 35-57 years, having high serum cholesterol levels. They were randomly divided into two groups and assigned either to drug therapy + dietary intervention program (restricting saturated fat + cholesterol intake) or drug therapy alone, for 7 years. The results revealed that the reduction in serum cholesterol levels in both the groups were comparable, indicating that restriction of cholesterol intake had no added advantage in lowering the serum cholesterol levels. Similar conclusions were drawn in LRCP studies for 7 years involving 3806 middle-aged volunteers.

How cholesterol is deposited in the arterial walls?

Cholesterol will not be deposited in smooth, undamaged arterial walls. It will flow freely in healthy arteries. But when the artery wall is damaged by any abrasive inflammatory materials like trans-fatty acids, excess blood glucose, rancid, oxidative materials like free radicals, certain food additives (chemicals) etc., LDLC & VLDLC, cholesterol will be deposited on the damaged arteries, form plaques and block the free blood flow. Sometimes blood clots may form over the plaques, resulting in total arterial block.

Elevated serum cholesterol is a complex physiological phenomenon.

Healthy arteries

↓

Inflammatory materials like trans-fatty acids, free radicals, excess free blood sugar, certain food additives (chemicals) & rancid oxidative materials act as abrasive material and cause damage to the arterial walls

↓

Blood LDL &VLDL cholesterol and other waxy materials will deposit on the damaged arterial walls & form plaques (cholesterol will not be deposited on healthy arterial walls)

↓

Blood vessels become narrow

↓

Blood clots may be deposited on plaques

↓

Total block of arteries & blood flow

↓

Causes CVD

After the arterial wall damage, as described above, the cholesterol, especially the LDLC and VLDLC, will be deposited over the damaged wall and block the free flow of blood, resulting in stroke and heart attack. Vegans and vegetarians may question, **why can't we reduce or stop consuming cholesterol? The simple answer is that the body can synthesize as much as 2000 mg of cholesterol per day, and dietary cholesterol is not essential for this deposition. Even vegans, who do not consume any cholesterol, will have normal or high serum cholesterol due to cholesterol biosynthesis, like others.** Hence, the causes for excess cholesterol biosynthesis and/or lower elimination have to be checked, as mentioned earlier.

How to reduce total serum cholesterol & bad LDLC/VLDLC?

- Persons having a family history (heredity) of hypertension, diabetes, hypercholesterolemia, CVD, and those having diabetes, kidney, heart and liver diseases, hormonal imbalance, must be more careful to control serum cholesterol levels.

- Avoid overeating and excess energy consumption, which result in obesity. Instead of having 2 or 3 heavy meals, consume more frequent (4 to 6) small meals, of which one must be multiple fruits and vegetable salads alone.

- Stay away from foods having trans-fatty acids. **Trans-fatty acids** are found in vegetable oils that have gone through hydrogenation in order to make them harder (saturated), such as margarine, vanaspathi, shortenings etc. They are also present naturally in butter, ghee and cheese, but they are not much harmful as that of TFA formed due to hydrogenation and prolonged over-boiling of oil during deep frying of chips and French fries etc., especially in restaurants. During the above process, the natural Cis-fatty acids will become trans-fatty acids, like elaidic, jucaric and vaccinic acids. Free radicals are formed due to rancidity. These TFA and free radicals in our foods are not at all good for our health. They are mainly found in refined processed junk foods made up of sugar, refined flour, margarine, butter, rancid fats and various food additives. Hence, avoid most of the bakery products, French fries, chips and sweets having the above items.

- Avoid rancid foods and repeatedly heated oils, which will have **free radicals/oxidative materials.** They will cause oxidative damage to many tissues, act as abrasive material and damage the arterial walls (blood vessels).

- **Avoid** further processed refined junk foods having several harmful food chemicals, sugar, refined flour, TFA, and oxidative free radicals, which will not only increase serum cholesterol, but also cause diabetes, obesity, cancer and other chronic diseases.

- Consuming anti-oxidants rich foods like **fresh** fruits and vegetables, vitamin E, C, organic selenium, pyrroloquinoline compounds, will help to limit the oxidation process, prevent the damage to the arterial walls and keep the cholesterol off the artery walls.

- Proper physical activities like exercise, swimming, cycling jogging/brisk walking are essential to maintain desirable body weight, BMI and keep cholesterol level under control.

- Consuming soluble fibers, which are abundant in green leafy vegetables, whole grains like brown rice, whole wheat products, oatmeal, vegetables and fruits. The liver will excrete body cholesterol through bile. Dietary fiber will bind with both endogenous and dietary cholesterol and excrete it from the body through stools.

- Probiotics and fermented milk products like curd, buttermilk, yogurt and mushrooms also reduce serum cholesterol.

- Spiller and Shipley (1977) concluded that gel-forming mucilaginous polysaccharides and other complex NSP like pectins, pentosans, gums etc. in the diet lower the serum cholesterol levels.

- Beynen and Liepa (1987) of Netherlands have concluded that glandless cottonseed protein has reduced the serum cholesterol levels in men.

- **Phytosterols are plant sterols or statins, which when consumed adequately (no RDA for it), reduces cholesterol synthesis in the liver, binds with cholesterol in the food as well as in the serum and eliminates cholesterol from the body.** Statins may also help the body to reabsorb cholesterol from built-up deposits on artery walls. **Some of the phytosterol rich foods are, cold pressed-katcha (not refined) oils, especially** sesame, peanut, rice bran, mustard and olive oils; unpolished grains, nuts, seeds, wheat germ oil, flax seed, peas, and various varieties of beans; vegetables like beets, Brussels sprouts, broccoli, cauliflower, onions and garlic. Some statins available in the market include atorvastatin (Lipitor), fluvastatin (Lescol), lovastatin (Altoprev, Mevacor), pravastatin (Pravachol), rosuvastatin (Crestor) and simvastatin (Zocor).

- **Avoid smoking totally.** Also avoid other tobacco products like snuff and chewing tobacco.

- Avoid or restrict alcohol consumption to less than 25 ml of pure ethanol (not more than 2 pegs or about 60 ml of 40% alcohol drinks like whisky per day).

- **Use oils and foods rich in MUFA and omega-**3 fatty acids (n-3 FA), like olive oil, flax seeds, fish oil, krill oil, chia seeds, spirulina, azola, canola oil, to supply 1 g of n-3 PUFA/day. Sufficient anti-oxidants, like selenium, vitamin-C &E are necessary, along with n-3 PUFA.

- Emotional stress produces compounds called "ceramides", which will cause internal clotting of blood and increase the serum cholesterol levels. So avoid emotional stress by leading a positive, contended, humorous life, doing yoga, meditation and breathing exercises.

- Fiber rich foods will reduce serum LDL and VNDL cholesterol levels.

How to increase good cholesterol (HDLC) level?
Just lowering the LDL cholesterol may not be enough for people at high risk of heart disease. Lower serum "bad" LDLC, along with higher level of "good" serum HDLC, will further reduce the risk of CVD. Although higher levels of HDLC can be helpful in reducing your risk of having a heart attack, researchers caution that you should also consider other risk factors for developing heart disease. It is possible that HDL may not be as helpful for some people as others, based on genetics, the size of the HDL particles and other proteins in your blood. If your HDL cholesterol level falls between the at-risk and desirable levels, you should keep trying to increase your HDL level to reduce your risk of heart disease. So to increase good HDLC:

- **Eat HDL boosting** n-3 PUFA rich foods like fish, fish oil, flax seeds (linseed)/oil, chia seeds, walnuts, hemp seeds, to supply 1000 mg of n-3 PUFA /day. Also consume HDL boosting foods like garlic, turmeric, ginger and fruits like guava, cranberries, red grapes etc. Most either have or contain antioxidants that give them the ability to lower LDL and increase HDL.

- **Avoid TFA and free radicals** rich foods, which will not only increase the bad LDLC levels, but also decrease the good HDLC. All artificial soft drinks, refined carbohydrates or white-flour products, sugar and hydrogenated fats containing foods like white bread, biscuits, cakes, doughnuts, burgers and many other bakery products, sweets and pastries must be avoided.

- **Use oils rich in MUFA (n-9FA) and Omega-3 PUFA** like olive oil, rice bran oil, peanut oil, mustard/canola oil, sesame oil, soya oil or blended oils having **SFA: MUFA (n-9): n-6 : n-3: fatty acids in a desirable ratio of 30:40:26:4 %.**

- Latest research has proved that short chain SFA like caproic, caprylic, myristic and palmitic acids, present in coconut oil, palm kernel oil, palm oil—especially coconut oil—at about 3-5 g levels in the diet, also elevates serum HDL levels. Based on this finding, the use of coconut oil has increased in western countries, especially in USA.

- **Exercise regularly:** Exercise is the key to every lifestyle-related disorder, be it heart disease or diabetes. Various studies have pointed out that aerobic and strength-training exercises have a positive impact on HDL levels in the blood. This is especially evident in case of obese women who follow a sedentary lifestyle. A study showed that resistance training (3 times a week) increased HDL by 15 percent in such women. Within two months of starting, frequent aerobic exercise can increase HDL cholesterol by about 5 percent in otherwise healthy sedentary adults. Your best bet for increasing HDL cholesterol is to exercise briskly for 30 minutes, five times a week. Examples of brisk aerobic exercise include walking, running, cycling, swimming, playing basketball and raking leaves—anything that increases your heart rate. You can also break up your daily activity into three 10-minute segments if you're having difficulty finding time to exercise.

- **Quit smoking:** Those who smoke are always at a greater risk of heart disease, due to increased cholesterol levels. A study by Forey BA and colleagues showed that participants who quit smoking had rapid, significant increases in HDL cholesterol. If you've been struggling to kick the butt for years, don't throw in the towel just yet—it truly is better late than never.

- Preferably, avoid alcohol. But those who are consuming alcoholic drinks, replace high alcohol content drinks like whiskey with **red wine** to a limited amount (<180 ml/day, with <13% alcohol). The reason experts recommend a moderate intake of red wine is because it is not completely bad for your health, particularly in people with high cholesterol. It is nothing but fermented grape juice, rich in **Resveratrol, Nirangenin and Lycopene, which will boost HDLC.** So limited intake of red wine (150 -180 ml /day) can actually boost your HDL by as high as 17 percent, according to a study. Europeans, who use olive oil for cooking, eat a lot of fish rich in n-3PUFA (EPA & DHA) and drink a glass of red wine regularly are having HDLC >60 mg/dl. Indians, Muslims and others, who are not accustomed to red wine, need not try this.

- **Lose weight.** Extra weight takes a toll on HDL cholesterol. If you are overweight, losing even a few kgs can improve your HDL level. For every 6 pounds (2.7 kilograms) you lose, your HDL may increase by 1 mg/dL (0.03 mmol/L). Maintain your BMI @ <24.

- **Statins. Phytostatins are plant sterols**, which block a substance your liver needs to synthesize cholesterol. This reduces cholesterol in liver cells, which causes the liver to remove cholesterol from blood. Many fruits and vegetables are rich in statins.

- **Avoid or restrict the use of** fatty red meats; crustaceans (shrimp & crab); full fat dairy products like cheese, whole milk, butter, and cream; hydrogenated fats like margarine, Vanaspathi and shortening, having high trans-fatty acids and saturated fat; processed meats like sausages; and bakery products like cakes, cookies and pastries and rancid foods. Fish and skinless chicken are preferred over red meat.

- **Calorie restriction:** Research on calorie restriction has found that moderate restriction of energy intake, especially of refined CHO origin, by 15- 20%, not only decreases your body weight, body fat, sugar and blood pressure, but also increases the blood HDL levels.

- **Herbs** like *Corus mas*, Red Yeast Rice (*Monoscus purpureus*), garlic, curry leaves, basil, holy basil (*oscimum sanctum*), white basil (*oscimum album*), turmeric, alfalfa, azolla, curry leaves, mint, oregano, dill, spirulina, rosemary, are rich in anti-oxidants and many more herbal active principals which will neutralize the free radicals and reduce the serum cholesterol levels, especially the bad LDLC and VLDLC.

In conclusion, we need not worry about the elevated serum cholesterol and their bad effects if we consume less than the recommended calories (1600-2200 Kcal. /day, depending on the age, sex and physical activity, as mentioned at several places in this book), do sufficient physical work, consume wholesome balanced diet, having no/least food additives and junk foods and minimize mental stress.

Chapter 8

Dietary Lipids—Fats and Oils

Lipids are organic substances soluble in fat solvents, but insoluble in water. This includes fats, oils, fatty acids, sterols like cholesterol and phytosterols, waxes, soaps, phospholipids, glycolipids and fat-soluble vitamins. However, the nutritionists took the last one to the category of vitamins because their functions are different from that of general lipids, except for solubility. During the process of digestion, all fats and oils will break down into fatty acids and glycerol. The glycerol will be utilized as a source of energy, just like any sugars.

What are oils and fats?

Fats are solids at room temperature, and will have more saturated fatty acids, while oils are liquids at room temperature and are made up of more unsaturated fatty acids. Oils come from many different plants and from fish. Fats are mostly of animal origin like lard, tallow and butter fat. However, the poultry lipids like emu oil, chicken oil and egg lipids will have more health promoting MUFA, and a few vegetable oils like coconut oil, palmolein and mohua oil are intermediate semi-semisolids. The melting point of a lipid depends on the fatty acid composition of it.

Commonly used cooking oils are canola, rapeseed, mustard oil, peanut oil, sesame oil, corn oil, cottonseed oil, palm kernel oil, palm oil, coconut oil, shea nut oil, safflower oil, soybean oil, sunflower oil, rice bran oil and olive oil. Food grade lard, tallow, butter, shortening and chicken oil are also used for cooking to some extent in Europe and Far East countries. Some oils and fats are used mainly as flavoring agents, such as walnut oil, butter fat (Ghee), almond oil, clove oil, cashew oil, fish oil and avocado oil.

Fatty acids

Edible fats and oils are mostly triglycerides or simple/ true lipids, made up of three molecules of fatty acids attached to one molecule of glycerol. Other lipids are more complex compounds, like phospholipids having phosphorous in it, glycolipids having CHO in it, derived lipids, waxes and sterols, like cholesterol. The fatty acids are broadly classified into **saturated** and **unsaturated** fatty acids. The saturated fatty acids are more stable, will have a common formula of $CH_3 (CH_2)_n COOH$, with no double bonds. On the other hand, unsaturated fatty acids will have one or more double bonds, with each double bond replacing two hydrogen atoms. The more the number of double bonds (unsaturation), the lesser the stability will be.

Figure 2. Structure of a fatty acid

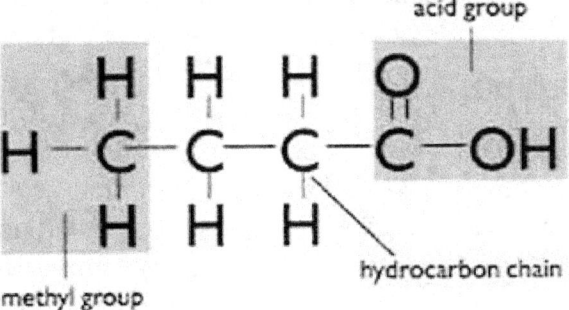

Saturated fatty acids (SFA) are acetic(C2), butyric(C4), caproic(C6), caprylic(C8), capric(C10), lauric(C12), myristic(C14), palmitic(C16), stearic(C18), arachidic(C20) and lignoceric(C24) acids, of which the stearic and palmitic acids are more common in fats and oils. The values in parentheses indicate the number of carbon atoms in each molecule of the fatty acid. SFA are not so bad, as many think, because they are more stable and protect the fat/oil from rancidity. Now many health authorities, including WHO and ADA are recommending 7-10% of the total calories from SFA origin. As such, a person who needs about 2000 calories per day can get 200 calories by consuming 22 g of saturated fats.

Unsaturated fatty acids

The unsaturated fatty acids have one or more double bonds (unsaturation) in their structure. If there is one double bond, the fatty acid is known as a **monounsaturated fatty acid (MUFA).** Examples are oleic and palmitoleic acids, of which the oleic acid is more abundant in all oils and fats, especially in olive oil, and to a lesser extent from canola (mustard/rapeseed) and peanut oil. In MUFA the double bond is at 9th carbon atom; hence, it is also called as n-9 fatty acid (omega-9 FA). If there is more than one double bond, then the fatty acid is known as a **polyunsaturated fatty acid (PUFA).** Linoleic acid is the most common PUFA found in oils which have two double bonds. The first double bond is between **n-6** and the next carbon atom; hence, it is also called as **n-6 (omega 6***)* fatty acid. Other **PUFA** are linolenic (**LNA**) or alpha LNA, eicosapenataenoic (**EPA**) and docosahexaenoic (**DHA)** acids. They are also called **n-3 (omega 3)** PUFA because the first double bond starts from n-3 carbon atom. They are heart, brain and arteries protective and they lower serum LDLC. The LNA, EPA and DHA have 3, 5 and 6 double bonds, respectively. LNA is abundant in flax seeds (linseeds), chia seeds, various nuts, spirulina, azola, canola (mustard/rapeseed) and soy oils; whereas the EPA and DHA are present in fish and krill oils and some marine algae. Other PUFA is arachidonic acid with four double bonds, but it is not an n-3 fatty acid; it is an n-5 FA.

Essential fatty acids (EFA)

EFA are fatty acids which cannot be synthesized by our body in sufficient quantity. Our body cannot synthesize fatty acids like alpha linolenic acid (n-3 PUFA) and linoleic acid (n-6 PUFA). Hence, they are dietary essential. From these fatty acids our body can synthesize others which are important for health. From linoleic acid, our body can synthesize oleic and arachidonic acids, and from alpha linolenic acid, our body can make EPA and DHA to some extent.

"*CIS*" and "*Trans*"-fatty acids

The unsaturated fatty acids occur as geometric isomers. Positioning of the double bond within the polyunsaturated fatty acid structure based on the arrangement of hydrogen atoms determines its type in one of the two ways. One arrangement is called *cis,* the other is called *trans.* Most of the natural fatty acids in oils are in the *Cis* form; whereas the *Trans*-fatty acids **(TFA)** were found naturally in ruminant fats, milk fat and tung oil. **TFA** can also be produced during hydrogenation of oils to make hydrogenated fats like vanaspathi, margarines, salad dressings and shortenings. Today, **trans**-fatty acids-free vanaspathi, margarines, salad dressings and shortenings are produced and marketed. TFA are also produced from **cis- FA (SFA, MUFA & PUFA),** during over boiling of oil at high flash point or repeated heating of oil for deep frying of foods in restaurants and fast food manufacturers. This conversion is more in case of PUFA rich oils like safflower, sunflower, corn and fish oils. Moreover, oils rich in PUFA without anti-oxidants will undergo rancidity on prolonged storage, resulting in release of free fatty acids and free radicals, which damage the arterial walls and causes atherosclerosis. The ***trans*-fatty acids** like elaidic, jucaric and vaccinic acids are **not good for health** because they will increase serum bad cholesterol (LDLC) and also cause abrasions to the blood vessels, resulting in damage to the arterial walls, platelet aggression and blocking of arteries and capillaries. Adequate dietary linoleic acid and antioxidants will reduce the harmful effects of TFA, to a considerable extent.

Oxidized fats/free fatty acids:

Prolonged storage, over boiling for a longer period, or keeping the oil in open containers for a longer period, will cause the oil to undergo oxidation and rancidity, resulting in release of free fatty acids (FFA). Presence of metallic ions like copper, nickel and zinc will catalyze the oxidation and bring rancidity at a quicker rate. Oils having more PUFA, like flax seed oil, fish oil, safflower oil, sunflower oil, corn oil and canola oil will undergo rancidity and oxidation at a faster rate than oils having lesser PUFA, like coconut oil and palm oil. Solvent extracted oils will undergo rancidity quickly, compared to cold pressed (Ghani pressed) virgin oils. Expeller oils will undergo rancidity at an intermediate rate.

Such rancid oils will lose their natural flavor and emit an undesirable odor and taste. Moreover, they are not good for health, due to free radicals in them. These free radicals cause cellular damage, Atherosclerosis, CVD, pre-mature ageing, cancer, asthma, arthritis, diabetes and many other chronic diseases. To overcome rancidity, antioxidants like BHT, BHA, Ethoxyquin, Santoquin, tocopherols are added at 1 kg/ton of oil. These antioxidants will scavenge on these free oxygen radicals and eliminate them from the body.

How are oils different from solid fats?

All fats and oils are a mixture of saturated fatty acids and unsaturated fatty acids. Solid fats contain more **saturated fats** and/or ***trans* fats** than oils. Oils contain more monounsaturated (MUFA) and polyunsaturated (PUFA) fats. Now the researchers have identified the exact role of each fatty acid in human health, as shown in **Table 8-1**. These findings have made the nutritionists revise the recommended lipid levels in a healthy diet.

Previously, the nutritionists were not distinguishing between O-6 PUFA and O-3 PUFA, so they were mostly recommending oils rich in O-6 PUFA like safflower, corn and sunflower oils. After distinguishing the role of these two PUFA and MUFA in human health recently, the dieticians in developed countries are now recommending oils rich in MUFA and O-3 PUFA.

Table 8-1: Role of fatty acids in human health and their sources

Fatty acid (FA)	Beneficial effects	Harmful effects	Major food sources
SFA- caprylic, caproic, lauric, myristic, palmitic & Stearic acids	More stable, do not undergo rancidity. 7 to 10% of dietary energy must come from SFA. Short chain FA are preferred.	Higher levels (>10% of dietary energy) increase TGL, LDLC & VLDLC	Body can synthesize from excess calories, butter, hydrogenated fat (vanaspathi), tallow, lard, coconut and palm oils
Palmitoleic, oleic acid (MUFA)	Increases good HDLC	Excess converted to stearic acid & increases TGL & LDLC	Olive oil, mustard oil, chicken fat, egg yolk, peanut oil, sesame oil
Linoleic acid (O-6 PUFA)	Reduces TC, B.P. LDLC, VLDLC, TGL	Rancidity, excess reduces HDLC, obstructive jaundice, gallstones, high requirement of vitamin A & E	Safflower oil, sunflower oil, corn oil
O-3 PUFA (LNA)	Reduces B.P, TGL, LDLC, VLDLC, cardio-protective, prevents thrombosis	High levels- rancidity, gallstones, high requirements of vitamins A & E	Linseed, chia, canola, rapeseed/mustard & soya oils, pearl millet, (bajra), human milk, various nuts

Trans fatty acids (elaidic, jucairic and vaccinic acids)	--nil-	Act as abrasive materials & damages arterial wall, forms arterial plaques, thrombogenic, increases LDLC, TGL	Partially hydrogenated fat, deep fried foods, especially chips & French fries, bakery products & oil rich foods made up of over-boiled oil, milk fat
Oxidized free fatty acids, free radicals	--nil-	- do - peroxidation, increase req. of vitamin A & E, may lead to cancer	All old, stored, prolonged deep fried & rancid oils

Functions of lipids:

Oils and fats form an integral part of our body, diet and nutrition. 6-20% of our body weight is fat. Fat, though much maligned, is an important part of our diet and serves many functions in our body. In rich developed countries, the fat/oil consumption is higher, supplying 35-42 % of dietary energy. So the dieticians and doctors in those countries are advising their people to reduce the fat calories to <30% of total calories. Ignoring these facts, dieticians in India and other poor Afro-Asian countries are also advising (wrong advice) their people to reduce the fat consumption to 25-30%, where it is already low at 12-17% fat calories.

- Lipids are concentrated sources of energy, supplying 9 calories/g, compared to 4 calories/g of proteins and CHO.

- Lipids impart palatability to the diet.

- Lipids impart satiety after eating. Lipids take a longer time for digestion and absorption; thereby, they suppress hunger and have low glycemic index. Hence, they are more suitable for diabetic patients.

- In a healthy diet, 25-30 % of total calories must be of lipid origin. For growing children, diabetic patients, athletes, pregnant and lactating women, the lipid calories must be 30-35% of total calories.

- Presence of fat in a diet is essential for the absorption of fat-soluble vitamins like vitamin A, D, E, K and other fat-soluble substances like carotenoid pigments present in the foods we eat.

- Apart from these functions, lipids supply essential fatty acids, which have vitamin-like functions in the body. These essential fatty acids are also important for the structure and function of cells in addition to supplying energy.

- Lipids are essential for integration of epithelial tissues, healthy skin, sebaceous glands, nervous tissues, liver and other tissues.

- ADA, AHA, CMFN, CNS, COMA, DHSS, ION, LRCP, NCCAAHA, NCEPHLBI and many health authorities have issued guidelines for reducing the risk of cardiovascular disease by dietary and other lifestyle practices. One of its general principles talks about reducing risks of CVD by reducing bad LDLC. The major food components that raise LDLC are trans-FA, rancid fats/oils, excess sugar, refined flours, saturated fats exceeding 10% of total calories and their combinations, especially associated with excess calorie consumption and sedentary lifestyle.

Table-8-2: AHA guideline for ideal fatty acid ratios for dietary lipids

Total fat intake	Maximum 30% of total calories supply
Saturated fats	Should be minimized to 10% of total calories or $1/3^{rd}$ of total lipid intake
Ideal MUFA(n-9): PUFA(n-6) ratio	1.5 :1 or n-6 must be 67 % of n-9
Ideal n-6: n-3 PUFA ratio	6:1 or n-3 must be 16% of n-6
Ideal SFA: n-9:n-6:n-3 ratio	27:41.5:27:4.5

Table-8-3: Fatty acid composition of commonly used fats and oils and actual human dietary requirements

Name of the oil or fat & human dietary requirements HDR)	Fatty Acids as % of Total Fatty Acids				
	Saturated Fatty Acids (SFA)	Mono Unsaturated Fatty Acids (MUFA)	n-6 Poly Unsaturated Fatty Acids (n-6 PUFA)	n-3 Poly Unsaturated Fatty Acids (n-3 PUFA)	Trans-Fatty Acids (TFA)
Human Dietary Requirements (HDR) as per AHA	27	41.5	27	4.5	Nil
HDR in Japan	28	43	23	6	Nil
Rice bran oil	21.0	41.5	36.0	1.5	--
Cotton seed oil	27.0	19.4	53.4	0.2	--
Linseed oil	10.0	19.0	15.8	55.2	--
Rapeseed oil	7.3	58.4	24.5	9.8	--
Canola oil	5.8	64.6	20.3	9.3	--
Mustard oil	6.3	63.8	22.6	7.3	--
Olive oil	21.0	72	7.0	--	--
Soybean oil	16.4	23.9	52.1	7.6	--
Sunflower oil	11.0	21.7	67.0	0.3	--
Safflower oil	9.9	16.3	73.6	0.2	--
Coconut oil	89.6	7.4	2.9	0.1	--
Peanut (groundnut) oil	20.1	49.3	29.8	0.8	--
Palm kernel oil	81.8	15.3	2.5	0.4	--
Palm oil	51.2	38.3	10.2	0.3	--
Shea nut oil	72	12	5	--	--
Sesame (gingelly) oil	13.8	41.0	44.8	0.4	--
Corn oil	14.2	27.5	57.3	0.9	--
Lard	41.7	44.5	10.9	0.9	--
Tallow	45.2	42.1	9.1	0.6	--
Chicken fat/oil	33.3	43.4	21.4	1.0	--
Egg yolk lipids	33.8	38.3	20.7	1.1	--
Fish oils	26.9	23.4	2.4	31.3	--
Butter	62.8	31.8	2.2	1.1	2.1
Hydrogenated fat (Vanaspathi)	90+	<7	<3	nil	3.4

The previous table indicates that none of the oils/fats has ideal fatty acid composition required for humans. However, some oils have fatty acids composition closer to the human recommendations. They are canola, rapeseed, mustard, peanut, sesame, rice bran and soya bean oils. However, in the canola, rapeseed and mustard oils, most of the MUFA is erucic acid and not oleic acid. On the other hand, linseed, safflower, coconut, palm, palm kernel oils, lard, tallow, milk fat and hydrogenated fat have highly deviated composition from the recommended ideal ratio.

Hence, for balancing the fatty acids, one has to consume a mixture of oils (one for the breakfast cooking, another for lunch and yet another for supper) or use a blending of oils, to get the ideal fatty acid composition in your diet. Studies at the National Institute of Nutrition as well as international research have shown that the blend plays a higher synergistic role than a single oil. For blending purpose, we can use canola, olive, peanut, sesame, coconut, palm or rice bran oils. Some combinations of blended oils are reported in **Table-8-4.**

Table-8-4: percent composition of some blended oils for ideal fatty acid composition

Names of oils	Formula 1	Formula 2	Formula 3	Formula 4	Formula 5
Flax seed oil	2%	3%	--	4%	--
Olive oil	28%	--	20%	26%	--
Rice bran oil	--	35%	--	--	30%
Canola/mustard /rapeseed /soy oils	40%	10%	60%	45%	30%
Coconut/palm oils	15%	15%	20%	25%	20%
Peanut/sesame oils	15%	20%	--	--	20%

How much oil do you need daily?

Fats and oils are an essential part of our food, but many people are afraid and over cautious in consuming lipid rich foods. A balanced diet for healthy living will neither ignore nor over prescribe lipid rich foods. Besides supplying essential nutrients like essential fatty acids, fat-soluble vitamins and phospholipids to the body, lipids are capable of supplying 2.25 times more energy than carbohydrates or proteins.

According to the American Heart Association, the optimum intake of fat for an adult is 30% of its total caloric intake. Therefore, an adult man requiring 2000 calories per day has to obtain about 600 calories (30%) from lipids. At a rate of 9 calories per gram of lipids, one has to consume about 67 gm of total fat per day. This 67 g includes both invisible (bound) and visible (added) lipids. Apart from visible fat/oil added during cooking, some amount of invisible fat is present in food items like cereals, pulses, nuts, milk, eggs, meat etc. as invisible fat. From the database generated on fatty acid composition in Indian foods and National Nutrition Monitoring Bureau diet surveys, the daily invisible fat intake is estimated to be 15 gm among the rural poor and 25 gm in the urban middle and high-income groups. Thus, the daily requirement of visible (added) fat/oil intake works out to be somewhere between 42 to 52 gm, depending upon physical activity and physiological status. However, in the average Indian diet, this added lipid level is far below this level, which is less than 35 g/day. Hence, Indian diets are deficient in lipids, especially essential fatty acids and fat-soluble vitamins.

This 67 g oil/fat must supply about 13 g of saturated fatty acids, 27 g of MUFA, 18 g of O-6 PUFA and 2 g of O-3 PUFA, and the remaining will be glycerol, lecithin, carotenoid pigments and other minor lipid fractions. Pregnant and lactating women and children need double the above quantity of O-3 PUFA for better growth of brain, nervous tissue and intelligence of the fetus/baby. Human milk, fish, fish oil, designer egg, pearl millet, linseeds (flax), chia seeds, soya, canola, rapeseed and mustard oil are rich sources of O-3 F.A.

This is one of the reasons for recommending mother's milk for babies.

Table-8-5: world consumption of different edible oils -2014

Oil source	World consumption (million tons)	Remarks
Palm oil	41.31	Most widely produced oil. Also used to make biofuel.
Soybean	37.54	Accounts for about half of worldwide edible oil production.
Rapeseed, mustard/ canola	18.24	One of the most widely used cooking oils in Europe, North India and North America
Sunflower	9.91	Common cooking oil, also used to make biodiesel.
Peanut oil	4.82	Mild-flavored cooking oil. Popular in India
Cottonseed	4.99	Major edible oil, often used in industrial food processing.
Palm Kernel	4.85	From the seed of the African palm tree
Coconut	3.48	Popular in Kerala (India), Sri Lanka & Philippines. Also used in cosmetics, mainly as hair oil
Olive oil	2.84	Used in cooking in Europe & in cosmetics & traditional oil lamps

- Besides the above oils, sesame, safflower, rice bran, shea nut, mohua oils are used for edible purpose. Castor oil, flax seed oil, cashew, almond, walnut oils etc. are used in cosmetics, pharmaceuticals, industries and as a top dressing for added flavor.

- The above figures include industrial, traditional lamps and animal feed use.

- Besides vegetable oils, animal fats like butter, ghee, lard, tallow, chicken fat, fish oils are also used for cooking, animal feeds and in industries.

How much oil are Indians and rest of the world consuming?

According to the above recommendations, at least 40 g of visible-added oil/person/day (excluding bound-invisible oil in various foods) is needed in a balanced diet. This comes to 14.6 kg oil per annum (12 kg/annum for obese/overweight persons and 15-24 kg/annum for growing children, sports persons, pregnant and breast feeding mothers). Based on the present population, India needs 18.25 million tons of oil/annum for cooking only. In India at least 10 % extra oil is used for traditional lamps in Hindu temples and houses and, another 5 % oil is used for industrial and animal feed uses. Hence, India needs around 22 million tons of oil/annum.

As per another statistical data, 18.9 MT of oil is used (for all purposes put together) in India during 2015, of which 13 MT are imported oil, mainly as palm oil, rapeseed oil and soya oil. Out of this 18.9 MT, 15% goes for non-edible purpose, as mentioned above. Hence, the per capita availability for edible purpose is a meager 16 MT, which works out to 12.8 kg/annum= 35 ml/day/person, one of the lowest in the world. On the other hand, the per capita oil consumption in developed countries is about 30 kg/annum; in developing countries it is 20 kg, and the world average is 26 kg. **As such, Indians are consuming a lipid and protein deficient diet, stuffed with diabetogenic CHO; resulting in more and more incidences of diabetes and CVD.**

Based on these data, it can be safely concluded that the oil consumption in India is only half of the world's average and supplies only 17.7% (male-female average) of lipid calories required, as against the recommended lipid calories of 25-30% of total calories. Ignoring these facts, our health authorities and dieticians are suggesting outdated "reduce oil consumption" (copying the Europeans and USA recommendations, for whom it still applies well), resulting in consumption of excess calories of CHO origin, leading to diabetes, obesity, CVD and many

more chronic diseases. So instead of recommending to reduce oil consumption, we have to recommend the reduction of total calories, especially of CHO origin.

Rice bran oil:

In recent years, rice bran oil has gained popularity in India, Japan and other Far East countries, due to its excellent health promoting properties. Rice bran oil is extracted from rice bran. It is very healthy because it has a MUFA-PUFA ratio close to the AHA recommend-dations. Moreover, rice bran oil has four powerful antioxidants, namely, gama oryzanol, tocopherols, squalene and tocotrienols. Oryzanol is unique for rice bran oil, which contains about 10,000 ppm of oryzanol. This makes rice bran oil a heart friendly oil and is called "Heart Oil" in Japan. Rice Bran oil provides a rich source of nutrition and also has a very promising role to play in, not only cardiac care, but also diabetes and other ailments. In olden days our ancestors consumed brown rice, which had great nutrition value due to its unique oil content. But in modern times we prefer polished rice, which is nothing but refined flour, having high glycemic index.

Table 8-6: Metabolic functions of active principles present in rice bran oil & other oils

Active principle	Functions	Remarks
Gama Oryzanol	Reduces total cholesterol & triglycerides. Has anti-carcinogenic, anti-itching & anti-dandruff properties	Rice bran oil is a very rich source of oryzanol
Tocotrienols	Powerful anti-oxidant, prevents rancidity & free radicals, retards progression of atherosclerosis & is an immune booster	Present in many oils, especially in cold pressed oils
Tocopherols & / Vitamin-E	Anti-oxidant, immune booster, reduces serum cholesterol, protects tissues from oxidative degeneration	---do---
Squalene	Maintains the tone of the skin	---do---

Body fat:

The amount of fat stored in adults of normal body weight ranges from 6-20 kg. This stored body fat will supply 50,000 to 200,000 K.cal. of energy, sufficient for several days of starvation. This stored fat also provides a large buffer capacity of energy balance in case of large deviations in energy supplied per day. However, this body fat is mainly SFA- stearic acid. Even though the energy is supplied from body fat during starvation, there will be deficiency of essential fatty acids and fat-soluble vitamins. Hence, regular dietary supplementation of recommended essential fatty acids and fat-soluble vitamins are essential for normal health. However, to prevent fat deposition, the daily total energy supplied through food shall not exceed the daily energy expenditure or requirement. Moreover, the energy expenditure and requirement decreases at the rate of about 1% annum after 50 years of age, mostly due to lesser physical activity.

Eat fat and get thin:

Dr. Mark Hyman (2016) of USA conducted studies in various universities with 6,000 volunteers interested in reducing the BMI and obesity. The volunteers were provided diets supplying 60% vs. 20 % of total energy from lipid sources, without increasing the total energy levels. Those who were consuming high fat diets were getting lesser calories (25%) from CHO, but normal 15% calories from protein sources. At the end of the study, Dr. Hyman noticed that those who were getting 60 % of the calories from lipids (+25% from CHO +15% from proteins) were thinner than those getting 20 % from lipids (+ 65% from CHO + 15% from proteins). He concluded that fat calories are safer than CHO calories. So, **"Eat fat and get thin."**

Chapter 9

Dietary Proteins

Proteins are made up of amino acids. During digestion, the dietary proteins will break down into various amino acids they have absorbed into the system. They are the building blocks of all animal tissues, including humans. Next to water, proteins are the major portion of our body, followed by lipids, minerals and very little CHO. Our body needs more than 24 amino acids for normal functioning of the body, growth, reproduction, repairs, wear and tear, synthesis of thousands of enzymes and to perform various metabolic functions in the body. Among them only nine are dietary essential, called **essential amino acids (EAA).** Others are non-essential amino acids. This doesn't mean that they are not needed. They are equally essential to the body, but they can be synthesized from EAA. Shown in **Table-9-1** is the list of EAA to be supplied through food for humans and their dietary source.

Table-9-1: Essential amino acids (EAA) and their major dietary sources

Name of the EAA	Major foods sources for these EAA (in the order of merit)
Histidine	Eggs, fish, milk protein, soy protein, meats, sesame, peanuts
Isoleucine	Eggs, fish, milk protein, soy protein, meats, various nuts & legumes
Leucine	Eggs, fish, milk protein, soy protein, meats, sesame, beans, nuts

Lysine	Eggs, milk protein, fish, meats, soy protein, various nuts & beans
Methionine	Eggs, fish, milk protein, sesame, meats, various nuts & beans
Phenylalanine	Eggs, milk protein, fish, soy protein, meats, peanuts, sesame, beans
Threonine	Eggs, fish, milk protein, meats, sesame, soy protein, beans, nuts
Tryptophan	Eggs, milk protein, fish, soy protein, meats, various beans, chia seeds
Valine	Eggs, fish, milk protein, soy protein, meats, sesame, beans, nuts

Functions of proteins:

- Nearly 18-22 % of our body weight is protein, depending on age, gender, BMI and food habits. Therefore, our body has to replace dead, damaged, wear and tear cells with new cells, using dietary proteins.

- All enzymes are made up of proteins. Our body will secrete thousands of enzymes to perform various normal physiological functions in the body. These enzymes are secreted, using dietary proteins.

- Proteins are needed for growth, reproduction, repairs and replacement of dead tissues with new ones.

- Protein deficiency in children causes diseases like marasmus, kwashiorkor, characterized by fatigue, underweight, limited growth, potbelly, cognitive development, poor mental health and more child mortality.

- Just like CHO, proteins will supply 4 K Cal. of energy/g, in case of dietary CHO and lipids deficiency.

- Excess dietary protein will be either utilized for energy release or stored as body fat, after deamination, depending on the need.

Protein sources:
Proteins are available both in plants and animals, but the proteins of animal origin have better digestibility, amino acid balance, higher biological value and protein efficiency ratio, as reported in the **Tables-9-2, 9-3a & 3b.** Table egg protein has the highest quality, followed by milk, fish, meat and various plant protein sources. Among plant proteins, rice and soya proteins have better nutritional quality, but in rice the protein level is low. Legumes like peas, chick peas, peanuts, all types of beans, sesame, flax, cashews, almonds, walnuts, hemp seeds, chia seeds, are rich sources of vegetable proteins. In general, all vegetable proteins are deficient in EAA, especially lysine and methionine. Hence, a blend of animal (especially eggs, fish and milk) and vegetable proteins in our foods offer a well-balanced dietary amino acid profile.

Table-9-2: Qualities of different protein sources

Foodstuffs	Biological value (BV)	Protein efficiency ratio (PER)	Net protein utilization (NPU)	Chemical score (CS)
Table egg	96	4.5	91	100
Milk	84	3.0	75	65
Fish	85	3.0	72	60
Meat	80	2.8	76	70
Soybean	64	2.0	54	57
Rice	64	2.0	57	60
Pearl millet	62	1.8	52	52
Chick pea	58	1.7	47	44
Finger millet	58	1.6	44	43
Peas	56	1.6	45	42
Peanuts	54	1.7	45	44
Wheat	58	1.7	47	42
Maize	45	1.3	34	35

Table 9-3a: Nutrients supplied by 100 g edible portion of different foods

Nutrients	Egg	Rice	Wheat	Milk
Protein (g)	13.3	8.5	10.0	3.3
Calories (K Cal)	162	346	352	65
Linoleic acid (g)	1.8	0.3	0.4	0.2
Cholesterol (mg)	40.0	0	0	20
Lysine (g)	0.96	0.43	0.31	0.32
Methionine (g)	0.54	0.22	0.16	0.10
Vitamin A (IU)	1180	3.3	106	117
Vitamin D_3 (IU)	70	--	--	0.3
Vitamin E (mg)	3	1.35	1.55	0.3
Vitamin C (mg)	0	0	0	2
Vitamin B_1 (mg)	0.4	0.21	0.45	0.05
Vitamin B_2 (mg)	1.0	0.16	0.17	0.19
Vitamin B_3 (mg)	0.1	1.9	5.5	0.18
Vitamin B_5 (mg)	1.4	1.2	1.3	0.35
Vitamin B_6 (mg)	0.13	0.24	0.57	--
Vitamin B_{12} (mg)	0.032	0	0	0.015
Folic acid (mg)	0.09	0.4	0.12	--
Choline (mg)	600	107	86	88
Biotin (mg)	0.08	0.01	0.005	0.04
Calcium (mg)	67	10	22	120
Phosphorous (mg)	240	65	102	90
Magnesium (mg)	60	20	18	68
Manganese (mg)	0.06	12	49	0.9
Sulphur (mg)	165	50	22	30
Zinc (mg)	43	2	15	3.6
Iron (mg)	43	3.2	4.9	2
Copper (mg)	0.08	1.0	0.8	0.04
Iodine (mg)	0.07	--	0.1	--

Table 9-3b: Nutrients supplied by 100 g edible portion of different foods (continued from previous page).

Nutrients	Soya	Fish	Lamb	Pigeon pea	Mung bean
Protein (g)	36.2	19.4	21.4	22.3	24
Calories (K Cal)	432	130	114	335	347
Linoleic acid (g)	10.0	0.5	0.2	0.4	0.4
Cholesterol (mg)	0	60	70	0	0
Lysine (g)	2.25	1.69	1.35	1.25	1.0
Methionine (g)	0.51	0.63	0.41	0.34	0.23
Vitamin A (IU)	711	--	--	--	63
Vitamin D_3 (IU)	--	--	--	--	--
Vitamin E (mg)	0.45	1.1	0.1	--	--
Vitamin C (mg)	--	6.8	0	0	0.0
Vitamin B_1 (mg)	0.73	0.06	0.15	0.32	0.42
Vitamin B_2 (mg)	0.39	0.08	0.25	0.33	0.20
Vitamin B_3 (mg)	3.2	0.85	5	3.0	2.0
Vitamin B_5 (mg)	1.6	1.6	1.3	--	--
Vitamin B_6 (mg)	0.22	0.22	0.03	--	--
Vitamin B_{12} (mg)	0	0.019	0.007	0	0
Folic acid (mg)	0.87	0.03	0.06	0.86	0.24
Choline (mg)	247	408	226	183	206
Biotin (mg)	0.03	0.05	--	--	--
Calcium (mg)	240	214	13	73	154
Phosphorous (mg)	230	280	173	101	127
Magnesium (mg)	25	10	15	24	16
Manganese (mg)	33	7	1.1	15	9.6
Sulphur (mg)	24	12	25	19	17
Zinc (mg)	15	30	11	53	30
Iron (mg)	10.4	34	20	2.7	38
Copper (mg)	1.1	6	1.1	1.0	9.3
Iodine (mg)	--	1.0	--	--	--

As per the RDA by many countries, a balanced healthy diet must supply about 0.8 - 1 g of protein/kg body weight/day for adults, depending on gender and age, and extra allowances must be given for growing children, athletes, pregnant women and breast feeding mothers. Moreover, in a balanced diet, at least one-third of this protein must come from animal protein sources like milk, meat, eggs and fish. As such, a person weighing 66 kg needs a minimum of 22 g of protein of animal origin, and the rest may be either from animal or vegetable protein sources. In developed countries, most of the dietary protein comes from animal protein sources rather than vegetable sources, because the animal proteins are cheaper than vegetable proteins in those countries.

To get this 22 g of animal protein, one has to consume about 200 ml milk (8 g) + 1 egg (6.5 g) + 30 g meat or fish (7.5 g) = 22 g protein. This works out to about 73 lit. of milk + 365 eggs + 11 kg meat per annum. However, the actual protein products consumption in India are 89 lit milk, a meager 57 eggs (after 10% export) and 5.1 kg meat (all meats put together) per capita, which supplies 9.7 + 1.0 + 3.3 = 14 g animal protein per person/day. This works out to 63% of the animal protein requirement. Hence, Indians are suffering from protein deficiency, especially from high quality animal protein.

Even the vegetable protein consumption in India and African countries is below the RDA levels, resulting in protein deficiency, and in children causing diseases like marasmus, kwashiorkor, characterized by fatigue, underweight, limited growth, potbelly, cognitive development as well as mental health and more deaths among children. This low protein consumption in India is not only due to poverty, but also due to growing vegetarianism (>40 % of Indians are vegetarians), ignorance, misconceptions and misguidance by our health authorities and religious holy persons. As per some definitions, if the average meat consumption is below 30 g/day, such persons are classified as vegetarians. Based on this statement, with just 14 g meat consumption per day, India is totally a vegetarian country. As such, average Indians are eating both total protein and animal protein deficient diets. Such low protein and oil consumption in India leads to excess consumption of CHO, leading to diabetes, CVD and other chronic diseases, as reported in FAO and ICMR documents.

Even though India ranks number one in milk production, on the basis of per capita milk consumption, it does not fall even within the top 100 countries. In the 100th ranking country, the milk consumption is about 100 kg/person/annum; whereas in India it is only 93 kg (89 lit.). On the other hand, the per capita milk consumption in Finland (number one country) is 362 kg. The per capita milk consumption in Sweden, Netherlands, Switzerland and Denmark is more than 300 kg/annum. In many other European countries, the USA and Australia, it is more than 250 kg.

Similarly, in egg production India ranks number three position, after China and USA, but the **per capita egg consumption is very low at 57 eggs (after 10 % exports) and falls in the bottom 10% countries, far less than the world's average and WHO's minimum recommendations**, as reported in **Table-9-5** following. On the other hand, the egg consumption in China, Mexico, Japan, Hong Kong, Czech republic and Spain is more than 300 eggs per annum, and in many other developed and developing countries it is more than the WHO's minimum recommended 183 eggs per annum.

Japanese researchers at Kyoto University have identified two compounds in eggs, namely, **lumiflavin and lumichrome,** which are capable of arresting the multiplication of cancer inducing viruses and also preventing normal cells from turning into cancerous cells. Moreover, egg is used as an antidote for several toxins and irritants consumed accidentally. It is especially good for gastric ulcer patients by protecting the mucous membrane of the stomach and for convalescent persons and tuberculosis patients for speedy recovery.

Indians consider milk as a vegetarian food and egg as a non-vegetarian food. Based on origin, both are animal foods and are best for all. **In fact, egg is more vegetarian than milk, as explained below**. Milk is a secretion of the udder after the calf is born, for feeding the calf (not for us by nature, but we are grabbing the milk meant for calf). Eggs are the secretion of ovary and oviduct. Once the hen matures, they produce almost one egg a day. So egg production in birds is just like menstrual cycle in women. Cocks are not needed for this secretion and egg production, even in the country hen in the free-range village side. If cocks are present, the egg is fertile. In the absence of cocks, only sterile, infertile eggs, having no life inside, will be produced. Hence, all farm (table) eggs sold in the market are lifeless, infertile eggs, irrespective of cage, cage-free, organic, free-range or range-fed. They will not hatch into chicks, even if you incubate them in the incubator or under a broody hen. If we don't eat such table eggs, they are going to be wasted and are not going to feed any chicks. Moreover, by consuming milk, we are grabbing the food of the calf. Hatching eggs (fertile eggs) are produced in breeder farms and are very expensive. Hence, there is no question of selling costly hatching eggs for table purpose.

Just like milk and eggs, even **honey is a food of animal origin**, produced by honey bees. Honey bees collect nectar (not honey) from flowers and store the nectar in their stomachs, where it will get mixed up with some enzymes, undergo biochemical changes and be converted into honey, which the bees will empty into the honeycomb chambers. Nectar has a very poor keeping quality, just like milk, but honey has the best keeping quality among all foods. It can be stored at room temperature for several decades.

All animals naturally depend on plants and other animals for their food. Even plants have life. By eating the grains and seeds, we are killing millions of plants, but we cannot survive without eating them. We can eat only lifeless table eggs, water and salt, but we and other animals cannot survive with these three alone. As long as we are eating foods of animal and plant origin for survival and not destroying them for fun, it is not a sin.

In spite of India's top position in kara-beef (buffalo meat) export and fourth position in broiler production, its positon in the meat consumption scenario is still worse, as shown in **Tables-9-4** and **9-5** following. **Among the 171 countries where the data is available on per capita meat consumption by FAO, India ranks as low as 167th, which is in the bottom five countries.** India's average annual meat consumption is 5.1 kg (11.2 lbs.) or 14 g/person/day, compared to 143 kg in Luxemburg, and more than 100 kg in Hong

Kong, USA, Australia, Austria, Spain, Cyprus, New Zealand and Denmark, as reported in **Table-9-4.**

In chicken meat consumption (**Tables-9-5 & 6**) also, with just 2.2 kg/annum, India ranks in the bottom 5% countries, even though India ranks fourth in broiler production. On the other hand, the chicken meat consumption in the top ranking country, Kuwait, is 97.5 kg. If the chicken is really harmful, what will be the fate of people in Kuwait and other countries, where the chicken meat consumption is more than 50 kg/annum? In fact, skinless chicken has < 3% fat, which is lower than that of cows' milk, chips, French fries and other deep fried foods. It is low in calories but rich in high quality protein and most of the essential minerals and vitamins. Moreover, **chicken meat is rich in serotonin, which reduces stress and keeps the person calm.** India's chicken consumption is far lower than the world average of 14.3 kg and even lower than Pakistan, Bangladesh, Sri Lanka and African countries' average.

In developed countries, as well as in many developing countries, most of their protein requirements are met from animal proteins. In fact, they get more calories from protein and oils, rather than CHO, as reported in earlier chapters. Even in very poor Afro-Asian countries, the meat consumption is far higher (5.9 to 9.3 kg) than in India. In many countries, the meat consumption is 10 to 30 times higher than in India. If meat and egg eating is the cause of hypercholesterolemia, then the incidences of hypercholesterolemia must be 10 to 30 times higher in more meat eating countries than in India, but this is not the fact. Actually, they enjoy better health, especially cardiovascular health, than Indians. These data have clearly indicated that there is no correlation between the cholesterol, egg and meat consumption and the incidence of cardiovascular diseases. There is no logic to argue that egg and meat consumption is the contributing factor for higher incidence of hyper-cholesterolemia and heart diseases.

The actual problem in Indian diet is protein and oil deficiency and excess consumption of refined CHO rich foods, excess calorie consumption, nutritionally imbalanced diet and fasting, based on the wrong guidance from health authorities, religious leaders and vegans, even though no such negative advice is given in any other country, where the meat consumption is 10 to 30 times higher and the egg consumption is 5 to 6 times higher than in India. **India is the best example for wrongful dietary advice on health and nutrition from copying the western countries' guidelines, where the situation is different.** As per the data available in 2015 from different authenticated sources like WHO, India has the fastest growing incidences of diabetes in the world. About 18.5% of the world's diabetics are in India, which will grow to 22% by the year 2020. The actual figure must be higher, because many millions of poor diabetic patients in rural areas are not included in this list.

Vegetable proteins lack several essential amino acids. Very poor performance of athletes in India and other developing South-Asian countries is not only due to their genetic background, but it is also due to protein malnutrition, imbalanced diets and wrong food habits. In African countries, their genetic background is more athletic, but poor nutrition and other non-nutritional causes are responsible for poor performance by their athletes. Other non-nutritional causes include lack of gyms, playgrounds, coaches and no encouragement from parents, teachers, politicians and public.

Table-9-4: Ranking of Countries based on Per Capita Meat Consumption - pounds/person/year

Country (by rank) MC-lbs.					
1	Luxembourg	314.6	10	Ireland	222.0
2	Hong Kong	295.9	11	Israel	219.8
3	**United States**	**279.1**	12	Bahamas	217.8
4	Australia	259.3	13	Macao	214.3
5	Austria	240.5	14	Canada	212.3
6	Spain	237.9	15	Netherlands Antilles	209.9
7	Cyprus	230.16	16	Slovenia	207.0
8	New Zealand	229.3	17	France	195.3
9	Denmark	222.0	18	Argentina	195.3

19	Saint Lucia	194.2	45	Chile	155.6
20	Italy	194.0	46	Uruguay	150.8
21	Czech Republic	190.9	47	Norway	144.8
22	Portugal	189.6	48	Grenada	144.2
23	Saint Kitts and Nevis	188.3	49	Slovakia	142.6
24	United Kingdom	185.0	50	Gabon	142.0
25	Iceland	184.5	51	Romania	140.9
26	Germany	183.6	52	Mexico	137.1
27	Belgium	181.7	53	Jamaica	134.9
28	Malta	181.7	54	Belarus	134.3
29	Serbia and Montenegro	180.8	55	Venezuela	134.0
30	Brazil	178.1	56	Brunei Darussalam	133.6
31	Greece	174.6	57	Estonia	131.6
32	Antigua and Barbuda	173.7	58	Mainland China	131.2
33	Taiwan	173.5	59	Panama	127.2
34	Netherlands	171.5	60	Latvia	126.8
35	Sweden	170.0	61	Kazakhstan	123.5
36	Poland	169.3	62	Lebanon	120.2
37	Saint Vincent and the Grenadines	169.1	63	Saudi Arabia	120.2
38	Barbados	161.8	64	Russian Federation	114.9
39	United Arab Emirates	159.6	65	Malaysia	113.1
40	Switzerland	159.4	66	Bolivia	113.1
41	Mongolia	159.4	67	Bulgaria	112.9
42	Dominica	157.0	68	Belize	108.5
43	Finland	156.1	69	Republic of Korea	107.8
44	Lithuania	155.6	70	Dominican Republic	105.2

71	Ecuador	102.5	98	Iran	67.0
72	South Africa	101.9	99	Namibia	66.4
73	Japan	100.1	100	Singapore	65.3
74	Suriname	100.1	101	Armenia	64.4
75	Turkmenistan	94.4	102	Seychelles	63.9
76	Mauritius	93.5	103	Libya	60.8
77	Trinidad and Tobago	92.2	104	Palestinian Territory	59.5
78	Albania	90.2	105	Thailand	58.9
79	Costa Rica	87.1	106	Botswana	57.3
80	Croatia	85.8	107	Peru	57.1
81	Ukraine	85.1	108	Tunisia	56.7
82	Moldova	84.2	109	El Salvador	54.9
83	Colombia	84.2	110	Guatemala	54.2
84	Republic of Macedonia	83.6	111	Uzbekistan	54.0
85	Guyana	81.4	112	Morocco	52.5
86	Honduras	80.5	113	Somalia	51.8
87	Jordan	80.5	114	Myanmar	50.7
88	Kyrgyzstan	76.9	115	Mali	49.4
89	Vietnam	76.9	116	Egypt	49.2
90	Timor-Leste	75.1	117	Sudan	48.5
91	Cape Verde	74.3	118	Bosnia	47.8
92	Swaziland	71.9	119	Algeria	47.6
93	Paraguay	71.2	120	Turkey	46.7
94	Mauritania	71.0	121	Congo	46.3
95	Cuba	69.7	122	Djibouti	46.1
96	Georgia	68.8	123	Nicaragua	44.8
97	Central African Republic	68.3	124	Syria	43.0

125	Azerbaijan	42.8	149	Niger	25.1
126	Maldives	42.8	150	Comoros	24.7
127	Angola	41.4	151	Ghana	23.4
128	Laos	38.8	152	Uganda	22.5
129	Yemen	37.7	153	Indonesia	22.0
130	Lesotho	37.7	154	Nepal	21.4
131	Zimbabwe	37.3	155	Liberia	20.9
132	Cambodia	36.2	156	Tanzania	20.9
133	Burkina Faso	35.1	157	Gambia	19.2
134	Kenya	34.0	158	Ethiopia	18.3
135	People's Republic of China	32.2	159	Guinea	16.5
136	Madagascar	31.3	160	Rwanda	16.5
137	Haiti	31.1	161	Iraq	15.7
138	Sao Tome and Principe	30.2	162	Sri Lanka	15.7
139	Afghanistan	30.0	163	Eritrea	15.7
140	Cameroon	29.8	164	Togo	14.3
141	Zambia	29.5	165	Bangladesh	12.8
142	Cote d'Ivoire	28.7	166	Mozambique	12.6
143	Guinea-Bissau	28.4	167	**India**	**11.2**
144	Chad	27.8	168	Sierra Leone	10.8
145	Senegal	27.3	169	Democratic Republic of the Congo	10.1
146	Benin	27.1	170	Malawi	10.1
147	Pakistan	26.9	171	Burundi	8.2
148	Tajikistan	26.2			

Table-9-5: Per capita chicken consumption & world ranking, curtesy – FAO, Rome

Country /area	Chicken- lbs./person/year	Ranking
Kuwait	214.5	1
Hong Kong	172.9	2
Israel	146.7	3
United Arab Emirates	130.1	4
Qatar	123.6	5
Brazil	105.2	6
Saudi Arabia	101.6	7
United States	**100.5**	**8**
Malaysia	82.2	9
Australia	78.3	10
Americas (N& S America)	77.7	--
Argentina	74.3	11
Chile	69.0	12
UK	68.4	13
South Africa	67.9	14
Venezuela	66.1	15
Canada	65.5	16
Mexico	65.5	17
Spain	64.9	18
Taiwan	61.7	19
Iran	54.7	20
Colombia	53.4	--
France	49.7	--
European Union	49.1	--
Europe	47.7	--
Russia	46.3	--
EU-27	39.2	--
Ukraine	37.9	--
World average	**31.2**	--
China	30.6	--
Asia average	20.5	--
Africa average	13.0	--
Sri Lanka	10.1	--
Pakistan	8.8	--
Bangladesh	5.7	--
India	**4.8 lbs.**	**Bottom 5%**

Table-9-6: Per capita egg & chicken consumption in some countries (USDA-2013 data)

Name of the country / area	Eggs per annum (Number)	Per capita chicken consumption/annum (kg)
World average	170	14.2
WHO- minimum recommendations	**183**	**11.0**
Asia	154	9.3
Africa	43	5.9
Europe	216	21.7
Americas	194	35.3
Argentina	126	35.4
Australia	138	38.6
Bangladesh	36	2.6
Brazil	146	47.8
Canada	204	30.0
China	**367(1st rank)**	**13.9**
Czech Republic	312	15.2
France	226	22.6
Germany	223	16.7
Hong Kong	**312**	**78.6 (2nd rank)**
India	**57(30% of WHO rec.)**	**2.2 (bottom 5%)**
Indonesia	102	6.3
Iran	148	24.9
Israel	**171**	**66.7 (3rd rank)**
Japan	**340 (3rd rank)**	**18.5**
Kuwait	**265**	**97.5 (1st rank)**
Malaysia	221	40,2
Mexico	**363 (2nd rank)**	**29.7**
Myanmar	77	18.6
New Zealand	171	32.4
Nigeria	65	1.9
Pakistan	48	4.0
Philippines	102	11.2
Russia	264	21.0
Saudi Arabia	102	46.2

South Africa	142	33.6
South Korea	287	14.1
Spain	324	29.5
Sri Lanka	48	4.6
Taiwan	267	28.0
Thailand	170	12.2
UAE	153	59.1
UK	196	31.1
USA	240	45.7
Vietnam	65	10.8

Based on the above data, it can be safely concluded that in many poor Afro-Asian countries, people are consuming imbalanced, poor quality foods, deficient in protein and lipids, due to poverty and ignorance. However, in India such poor quality imbalanced food consumption is not only due to poverty and ignorance but also due to misbeliefs and misguidance by our outdated health professionals, religious leaders and vegans. Therefore, even affordable middle and high income group Indians are consuming imbalanced foods, deficient in lipids and proteins, leading to consumption of high CHO foods and resulting in more incidences of diabetes, obesity, CVD and many other chronic non-infectious diseases.

Chapter 10

Micronutrients

Micronutrients are essential nutrients for the body, just like macronutrients (CHO, lipids & proteins), but are required in small quantities, in milligrams or micrograms. However, they are as important as macronutrients, because they play a vital role in the body metabolism, enzyme system, various physiological functions, reproduction and growth. Micronutrients as part of various enzymes, coenzymes, cofactors etc. perform several physiological functions in the body. They are needed for optimal growth rate, reproduction, health, immunity and overall health of the individual. At the same time, they cannot be synthesized in the body. Hence, their dietary supplementation is very essential. Their deficiency will produce certain deficiency diseases. **All minerals, vitamins and some other herbal active principles, or phyto-chemicals, come under this category.**

Vitamins are organic substances, whereas minerals are inorganic substances. Vitamins are either water-soluble or fat-soluble substances, depending on their solubility in water or fat solvents. Fat-soluble vitamins are A, D, E and K. The water-soluble vitamins are the B-complex group of vitamins, like B-1,2,3,4,5,6,7,8,9,12, B-15, and vitamin-C, or ascorbic acid. These vitamins' requirements, their functions and toxicity are indicated in **Table-10-1**. The recommended RDA and dietary requirements of nutrients vary from country to country, and within the country, by various authorities, like ADA, AHA, USDA, NRC, NIN, WHO etc.

Dietary minerals or elements are classified based on their quantity (RDA) required by humans. They are macro minerals, trace minerals and ultra-trace minerals, or elements. The macro minerals are required in large quantities, in grams; trace minerals are required in milligrams; and the ultra-trace minerals are required in micro grams, but all are dietary essential and play a major role in the body's metabolism and health. However, some ultra-trace minerals may be available naturally in different foods. Examples of macro or major minerals are calcium, phosphorus, magnesium, potassium, sodium, chloride and sulphur. Trace elements are manganese, zinc, iron, copper and iodine. Ultra-trace elements are selenium, cobalt, chromium, molybdenum, fluorine, boron, silicon etc.

Is it necessary to take the supplemental micronutrients daily?
Fat-soluble vitamins and all minerals will be retained in the body, stored in the liver, bones and other tissues for a longer period. Hence, if higher than the RDA is consumed in a day, further daily supplementation is not needed for several days, maybe up to one month. However, it is advisable to take RDA levels only on a daily basis instead of consuming large quantities at a single time, because higher doses will be toxic. The water-soluble vitamins will be excreted from the body within a short period, maybe in few days. Hence, daily consumption at RDA levels or below is recommended if the food consumed is not balanced.

If you consume a balanced diet, containing 150-250 g fresh mixed fruits, 200-250 g fresh multiple vegetables, including green leafy vegetables, 300-400 ml 2% milk or milk products, 1 egg, 50 g fish, 50 g lean chicken meat, (for vegetarians/vegans = 100-150 g lentils/beans/peas/nuts/tofu etc.) and 150-300 g of whole multiple grain products daily, depending on the age, gender, body weight and physical activity, there is no need for daily supplementation of vitamins and minerals in the form of tablets. However, supplementation is needed for growing children, pregnant and lactating women, patients, convales-cents and sports persons. However, even this supplementation

is not needed at RDA levels because some nutrients will be available in the regular foods itself.

Table-10.1: Functions, Requirements (RDA) & Deficiency Symptoms of Micronutrients (vitamins & minerals)

Micro-nutrients & RDA	Functions	Deficiency Symptoms	Toxicity
Vitamin—A 5000 IU	Vision, reproduction, immunity, growth, epithelial & mucosal tissue health	Xerophthalmia, poor growth rate, low fertility rate, abortion, low disease resistance, ataxia	Hyper pigmenta-tion,fatigue, vertigo
Vitamin-D3 -400 IU	Calcium & phosphorus utilization, bone & teeth mineralization	Fragile bones, bowed legs, poor growth rate & rickets-beading of ribs	High blood calcium, calcifi-cation of soft tissues
Vitamin-E -30 IU	Immunity, reproduction, anti-oxidant, neuro-muscular transmission	Muscle weakness, low fertility, encephalomalacia, premature birth	Interferes with vitamin K, hemorr-hages
Vitamin-K -80 mcg	Blood coagulation, arrest bleeding	Internal & external hemorrhages	Jaundice
Vitamin-C -75 mg	Better immunity & heat tolerance, anti-oxidant, alleviates stress	Scurvy, breakdown of immunity, bleeding gums, heat strokes & stress	Abdominal cramps, nausea, diarrhea
Thiamine-B-1 -1.7 mg	Intermediate metabolism, appetite, health of nerves	beriberi, anorexia, hypothermia, oedema	—
Riboflavin -B-2 -1.7 mg	Cell respiration, growth	Gingivitis, ulcers at mouth, corners & tongue photophobia	—
Niacin-B3- 20 mg	Coenzyme-NAD, carbohydrate metabolism	Pellagra, dermatitis, poor growth rate	Vasodila-tation, dizziness, nausea

Choline-B4 -400 mg	Coenzyme, lipotropic agent, prevents fatty livers, neuro-transmitter, methyl donor	Fatty livers, poor growth rate, lack of muscle coordination	Tension, headache
Panto-thenic acid -B5-10 mg	Coenzyme-A, metabolism of CHO, lipids & protein	Dermatitis at corners of mouth, eye & feet, abortion	—
Pyridoxine -B6- 2 mg	Protein metabolism, growth, convert tryptophan to niacin, nervous health, coenzyme	Anemia, anorexia, growth depression, convulsions	Neuro-pathy, ataxia, photosen-sitivity
Biotin-Vitamin-H, or B7- 300 mcg	Lipid & protein metabolism, growth, coenzyme	Dermatitis at corners of mouth, eyes & feet, nausea,	—
Inositol-B8 -40 mcg	Nucleic acid & RBC formation,	Anemia, fatty liver, <growth, convulsions	—
Folic acid-B9-400 mcg	Metabolism, growth, blood formation	Anemia, growth depression,	Masks B-12 deficiency
Cynacob-alamine-B-12-6 mcg	Cofactor, nucleic acid formation, nerve health blood formation	Poor growth, anemia, fatty livers nervous symptoms,	—
Dimethyl-glycine-B-15	Increases muscle energy, anabolic	Poor muscle power	—
Calcium – 1000 mg	Bone & teeth, blood clotting, neural transmission	Rickets, fractures, prolonged blood clotting time	Calcification of soft tissue
Phosphorus-1000 mg	--do--, nucleic acid, phosphorylation, coenzyme	Neuromuscular, renal & skeletal disorders,	Hypo-calcemia
Magnesium 400 mg	phosphorylation, coenzyme, nerve impul transmitter	Muscular tremors & convulsions	Diarrhea, Hypo-calcemia
Sodium-2400 mg	Acid base balance, osmotic pressure, muscle function	Dizziness, exhaustion, Respiratory failure, apathy	Hyperten-sion, nausea, tissue dehydration

Potassium- 3500 mg	---do---, cardiac muscle function	Muscle weakness	Excess tissue hydration
Chloride -3400 mg	Acid base balance, gastric HCl production, osmotic regulation	Impaired osmotic pressure, gastric digestion Impaired	—
Sulphur -300 mg	Spares methionine, metabolism of proteins	Impaired growth	—
Manganese -2 mg	Forms organic matrix for bones & teeth, enzymes- energy metabolism, prolidase	Poor bone mineralization, ataxia, immunosuppression	Psychiatric & Neurological disorders
Zinc-15 mg	Carbonic anhydrase & other enzymes, immunity, insulin production	<growth, hair loss, dermatitis, poor immunity	Gasto-intestinal upset, vomiting, sweating
Iron-18 mg	Prosthetic group for many enzymes, electron transport, RBC formation- part of hemoglobin	anemia, anorexia, Irritability, lethargy	Haemo-chromatosis, Haemosi-derosis
Copper -2 mg	Coenzyme-A, uricase, RBC formation, immunity	anemia, ataxia, spastic paralysis	Liver damage
Iodine -150 mcg	Thyroxine production, controls BMR, thermoregulation	Goiter, <reproduction <growth	Hyper-thyroidism
Selenium -70 mcg	Immunity, spares vitamin-E, glutathione peroxidase, anti-oxidant	Muscular dystrophy, immune-deficiency, pancreatic dystrophy	—
Molybde-Num -60 mcg	Xanthine oxidase, DNA & RNA synthesis	Poor growth rate	gout
Chromium -120 mcg	Insulin, poor glucose tolerance	Poor growth rate, Diabetes	—
Cadmium	Suppress cholesterol synthesis	—	—
Cobalt	Part of vitamin-B-12	anemia , poor fertility	—
Fluorine	Bone & teeth strength	—	Bowed legs, teeth discoloration
Boron	Integrity of cell walls	—	—

Synergism and antagonism among micronutrients:

Synergism and antagonism exist among many nutrients and non-nutrients, especially among vitamins and minerals. Synergism is like compatibility and antagonism is like incompatibility. If synergism exists, their requirements decrease. On the other hand, antagonism will increase their requirements. In general, there is antagonism among fat-soluble vitamins. For example, excess of vitamin-A, will increase the requirement of other fat-soluble vitamins. Oxidized-rancid lipids will increase the requirements of fat-soluble vitamins. Synergism and antagonism among micronutrients are reported in **Table-10-2.**

Table-10-2: Synergism and Antagonism among vitamins and minerals:

Nutrient	Synergism with	Antagonism with
Vitamin-A	Carotenoid pigments	Vitamins- E, D, K, oxidative rancid lipids
Vitamin-D	Calcium	Vitamins-E, K
Vitamin-E	Selenium	Vitamins- A, D, K, oxidative rancid lipids
Vitamin-K	—	Vitamins- A, D, E, Anti-coagulants
Vitamin-C	—	Vitamin-B-12
Vitamin-B1	—	Amprolium (anti-parasitic drug)
Choline -vitamin B4	Methionine, betaine	---
Vitamin-B12	Cobalt, Folic acid	Vitamin-C
Calcium	Vitamin-D, lactose, citric acid	Phosphorus, magnesium, Phytates, oxalates, fluorine
Phosphorus	Potassium	Calcium, magnesium, aluminum
Magnesium	—	Calcium
Potassium	—	Sodium
Sodium	—	Potassium
Copper	—	Zinc, molybdenum, iron
Iron	—	Copper
Molybdenum	—	Copper
Zinc	—	Copper
Lysine (essential amino acid)	—	Arginine (essential amino acid)
Arginine	---	Lysine

Extra-nutritional functions of nutrients:

Besides the above nutrition related functions, micronutrients perform some additional functions in the body. The dietary requirements of them to perform these additional functions are usually higher than the normal requirements. These additional functions are mainly immunomodulatory and anti-oxidant functions. These immune modulators will boost the general immunity, prevent break down of immunity due to stress, toxins and diseases, prevent vaccination failure, act as anti-stressors, anti-oxidants, tonics, toxin neutralizers, anti-viral agents and rejuvenate the immune system in the body, as shown in **Table-10-3.**

Nutrient	Extra-Nutritional functions
Proteins	B-cell immunity function debilitated, atrophy of thymus
Arginine	Augments T-cell response, reduces hypertension, quick wound healing
Lysine	Check viral proliferation, prevents fatty livers, muscle building, immunity
Omega-3 fatty acids	Increase the concentration of T-cells and cytokines, increases HDLC
Vitamin-A	WBC synthesis, invasion of macrophages to kill microbes, protects mucus membrane and epithelial tissue, prevents certain types of cancer
Vitamin-E	Powerful anti-oxidant, production of interleukin-2, which kills microbes and cancer cells
B-complex	RBC & WBC production, intermediate metabolism, cell mediated immunity
Choline or Vitamin-B-4	By controlling homocysteine production, it controls CVD
Vitamin-C	Powerful anti-oxidant, prevents stress, anti-viral, killer cells, lymphocytes & interferon production
Manganese	Macrophage activity, enhances natural killer cells, immunity booster

Zinc	Prevents Immunodeficiency diseases and certain forms of cancer. Impaired thymus function, WBC production, serum IgM production, plaque forming cell response
Iron	Blastogenic response, circulating T-cells, humoral immunity antigen specific antibody titre, lactoferrin production, which invades microbes
Copper	T-cell controlled infections, T-cell mitogen response, phagocytic cell anti-inflammatory effect
Selenium	Powerful anti-oxidant, production of cytokines, prevents virus multiplication, especially influenza virus
Chromium	WBC respond to fight infection

Newly added vitamins/micro-nutrients:

As science progresses, newer micronutrients/vitamins are added to the list. They will perform several vital functions in the body, especially in metabolism, disease resistance and also work synergistically with other nutrients i.e. boosts the action of other nutrients. Their deficiency: may not show any significant deficiency symptoms. However, if they are present in sufficient quantities, they will improve disease resistance, metabolism, eliminate toxins, protect vital organs from damage and so on. Now choline chloride or simply called choline has been included in the list of water-soluble vitamin-B complex group, as vitamin-B4. Another chemical, known as dimethyl-glycine, has been added to the vitamin-B complex group as vitamin-B-15. This will increase the muscular energy, improve the muscle power and act as an anabolic, suitable for athletes to build muscular power. It is not a banned drug, like steroids.

Choline is a vitamin-like essential nutrient and a methyl donor involved in many physiological processes, including normal metabolism and transport of lipids, methylation reactions, and neurotransmitter synthesis. Now it is included as one of the B-complex group of vitamins, as vitamin-B-4. Choline deficiency causes muscle damage and abnormal deposition of fat in the liver, which results in a condition called non-alcoholic fatty liver disease.

Choline spares other methyl donors in the foods, namely, methionine and betaine. Genetic predispositions and gender can influence individual variation in choline requirements and thus the susceptibility to choline deficiency-induced fatty liver disease. The recommended adequate intake (AI) of choline is set at 425 milligrams (mg)/day for women and 550 mg/day for men. Choline is involved in the regulation of homocysteine concentration in the blood through its metabolite betaine. By this act, choline prevents CVD.

Besides the micronutrients listed in Tables 10-1, a new list of herbal active principles, which have some specific functions in the body, is presented in **Table-10-4.** Since many of these principles have antimicrobial activities, they can be used as alternative to antibiotics. They can also be used for boosting the immunity in the body and disease resistance.

Table-10.4: Recently identified active principles present in foods, which will improve the overall health & performance, similar to other micronutrients

Active Principles	Effects In The Body
Sialic acid	Anti-microbial, anti-inflammatory, anti-viral and, performance enhancer
Lecithin	Conjugates with vitamin-B12 & prevents Alzheimer's disease, nervine tonic, emulsifier, helps in fat digestion
Phosvitin	Anti-oxidant, nervine tonic
Lumiflavin, Lumichrome	Anti-oxidants, anti-carcinogenic, skin and retinal tonic
Lysozyme	Anti-microbial, immune booster
Intralipid	Carrier for fat soluble vitamins and drugs , reduces LDLC
Sulphoraphane	Anti-carcinogenic, immune booster
Taurine	Retinal tonic, prevents atherosclerotic plaque formation &CVD
Betaine	Methyl donor, prevents atherosclerotic plaques formation& CVD, controls diarrhea
Eugenol, Eugenic acid	Immunomodulators

Carotenoids, Lutein	Antioxidants, anti-cancer agents & retinal tonic
Lycopene,Nirangenin, To Cotrienols	Lowers bad cholesterol-LDLC
Phytosterols-Statin,	Increases good cholesterol-HDLC & decreases bad (LDLC)
Quercitin,Luteolin, Diosgenin, Citogenin	Stimulates insulin secretion and controls diabetes
Gamma Oryzanol	Increases HDLC & anti-oxidant

Probiotics or direct fed microbials (D.F.M.):

Probiotic is a live microbial food supplement, which beneficially affects the host by improving its intestinal beneficial microbial balance, resulting in a healthy gut, production of certain nutrients like vitamins-K, B12, and checks the growth of harmful microbes like E.coli and salmonella. Probiotic preparations are made from stable cultures of bacteria, yeast and fungi. Commonly included probiotic preparations in various combinations are:

- Bacteria: Strains of *Lactobacillus, Leuconostoc, Bifidobacterium, Pediococcus* and *Streptococcus*

- Fungi: Strains of *Aspergillus*

- Yeast - Strains of *Saccharomyces.*

Probiotics benefit the host by,

i) Having a direct antagonistic effect against specific group of undesirable or harmful organisms through the production of antibacterial compounds and eliminating or minimizing their competition for nutrients

ii) Altering the pattern of microbial metabolism in the gastro-intestinal tract

iii) Stimulation of immunity

iv) Neutralization of enterotoxins produced by pathogenic organisms

In general, probiotics replace antibiotics and their ill effects without any side effects, improve the overall health status of individuals, maintains better gut health and improves the disease resistance power of individuals.

Chapter 11

Food Additives

Food additives are chemicals added to the foods during processing/cooking to improve their consumer acceptance, in terms of color, consistency, flavor, taste, texture, eye appeal, crispiness, keeping quality, customer attraction, and convenience to handle and transport. Many food additives are harmful to the health when consumed for a length of time. Today, almost all refined foods, packaged foods, restaurant foods, and fast foods contain several food additives, creating several health hazards, which can be curtailed by avoiding them.

Until the end of 19th century, the term food additives did not exist. Only natural products like salt, sugar, yeast, sodium bicarbonate, vinegar and few natural pigments were present in food products, and the foods made with them were not only tasty, but also healthy. Even a few decades ago, only very few food additives were available in the market.

Now the food additives industry has grown beyond boundaries into a mega industry, producing **not hundreds**, but several **thousands** of varieties of food additives. These additives include preservatives, used to prevent or inhibit spoilage of food by microorganisms, acidifiers, buffers, colors, color enhancers, color retention agents, sweeteners, milk substitutes, flavors, flavor enhancers, flavor retention agents, conditioners, taste enhancers, acidity regulators, anti-caking agents, antibiotics, emulsifiers, mold inhibitors, stabilizers, thickeners, sweeteners, gelling agents and many more, as described in **Table-11-1**. There are several thousand food additives in the market today, and writing all about them is beyond the scope of this book. Hence, only a few examples are mentioned in this table.

Table-11-1: Food additives commonly used in junk/fast foods

Type of food additive/purpose of addition	Examples of chemicals under each category
Acidifiers, organic acids, which add "sharper" sour taste and flavors to foods, also act as preservatives & mold inhibitors	Acetic, benzoic, citric, propionic, tartaric, malic, formic, fumaric and lactic acids, vinegar,
Acid regulators- maintains pH, acts as buffers also	Adipates, calcium acetate, calcium gluconate, lactones, magnesium sulphate, carbon dioxide
Alkalizers – increase the pH of the foods, helps in fermentation, baking	Baking soda (sodium bicarbonate), potassium bicarbonate, calcium carbonate, ammonium carbonate
Anti-caking agents- keep powders from caking or sticking together	Aluminum silicates, silicon dioxide, silicates, kaolin, magnesium carbonate/oxide/silicate/phosphate, dicalcium phosphate polyphosphates, bentonite, calcium carbonate, stearic acid, talcum powder
Anti-oxidants- prevent oxidative rancidity & spoilage of foods, especially lipids, also act as preservatives for lipids	Butylated hydroxyl anisole (BHA), Butylated hydroxy toluene (BHT), santoquin, ethoxyquin, vitamins C & E, ascorbyl palmitate, ascorbyl stearate, tocopherols, propyl gallate, citric acid,TBHQ, tertiary-butyl-hydroxy-quinone(TBHQ), Dilauryl-thio-dipropionate (DLTDP), dodecyl gallate, selenium, dilauryl thiodipropionate
Antibiotics- **(synthetic)** prevent microbial spoilage of foods.	Nisin, natamycin, neomycin (both are banned)
Antibiotics- anti-microbial-anti-viral-antiseptic **(natural)**- herbs & spices	Garlic, turmeric, honey, lysozyme (found in egg white), apple cider vinegar, extra virgin coconut oil
Anti-foaming agents reduce the foaming in	Poly-dimethyl-siloxane (PDMS), polyethylene glycol-8000, silicon glycol,

foods, especially oils during deep frying	flurosilicons, polyphopylene, polyacylate
Foaming agents increase the volume, by incorporating air, brings frothiness	Egg white, soaps, whole milk powder, sodium lauryl sulphate (SLS)
Buffers- used to control the acidity and alkalinity of foods	Potassium citrate, sodium citrate, calcium phosphate, poly phosphates, adipates, calcium acetate
Bulking agents-increase the bulkiness of the food	Starch, carboxy methyl cellulose (CMS), sodium laural sulfate (SLS)
Bleaching agents	Chlorine, hydrogen peroxide, ozone, chlorine dioxide
Chelating agents-improve the activity and bio-availability of the product	Ethylene di-amino tetra acetic acid (EDTA)
Coloring agents- give attractive color to the foods- (there are hundreds of food colors)	Amaranth, annatto, anthrocyanin, carotene, astaxanthin, allura red, beet red, bixin, black-PN, brilliant green, brilliant blue, caramel, capsanthin, chocolate brown, carmisine, chlorophyll, erythrosine, iron oxide, lutein, sunset yellow, tartrazin, vegetable carbon, yellow-2G, zeaxanthin
Color fixing agents- fixes **color** to the food uniformly	Potassium nitrate, potassium nitrite, sodium nitrite, ferrous gluconate, ammonium nitrite
Color retention agents- prevent loss of color during cooking, storage etc.	Nicotinic acid, polyvinyl-poly-pyrollidone, ferrous gluconate, vitamin B3 (niacin), stannous chloride
Deodorants- remove undesirable odor from the foods & keep them fresh	Activated carbon, activated charcoal, cardamom, clove oil, essential oils, cinnamon oil
Emollients- seasoning oils-reduce irritation by other food additives or by the food itself	Coconut/olive/almond oils, coco butter
Emulsifiers- keep water & liquid well mixed together in an emulsion form	Polysorbates, lecithin, ammonium phosphatides, CMC, pectins, alginates, egg yolk, lecithin, tannin, agar, calcium tartrate
Enzymes- reduce the toughness of the foods	Yeast, papain, bromilin, ficin, cellulose, hemi-cellulase
Flavoring agents- give attractive aroma to the foods-there are	Asafetida, cardamom, cinnamon, mint, vanilla, many spices, fruit essences, onion, rose essence, meat extracts, essential oils

innumerable flavoring products	
Flavor enhancer- enhance the flavor of the foods, works in association with flavoring agents	Monosodium/ ammonium /potassium-glutamate (MSG or ajinamoto), Ca-5-ribonucelotide, ethyl maltal, dipotassium-guanylate, dipotassium inosinate, leucine, glycine, magnesium digluconate, glutamic acid
Flavor retention agents- retain flavor/aroma for longer period, until consumption	Amylases, calcium sulphate, L-cystine, chlorine dioxide, amylases, sodium succinate
Firming agents- keep the products firm & reduce friability	Magnesium sulphate, calcium citrate, tannins, gum tragacanth,
Foaming agents- increase the volume, by fixing air bubbles in between	Live yeast, egg white powder, eno, fermentation agents, soaps, SLS, CMC
Gelling agents- give the product a firmer texture, also act as binders	Gelatin, agar, gum tragacanth, guar gum, locust bean gum, gluten, wheat germ oil, carrageenan,
Glazing agents- provide an attractive shiny appearance or protective coating to foods	Bees wax, shellac, camellia wax, carnauba wax, paraffin
Humectants-prevent foods from drying out	Glycerine, isomalt, lactitol, maltitol, mannitol, polydextrose
Leavening agents- used in bakeries	Baker's yeast, sodium bicarbonate, mandarin oil, probiotics
Mineral salts- used to improve/alter taste	Rock salt, black salt, calcium chloride /phosphate, ammonium hydroxide, magnesium sulphate,
Mold inhibitors- cum-preservatives	Sodium benzoate, potassium sorbate, citric acid, formaldehyde, potassium sorbate, activated carbon/charcoal, many organic acids and their salts
Preservatives- prevent or inhibit spoilage of food by microorganisms; there are several hundreds, having some other functions also	Benzoic acid, citric acid, other organic acids, salt, smoke, sulfites, sugar, formaldehyde, sodium benzoate, sodium metabisulfite, sorbates, boric acid, borax, EDTA, ethyl paraben, propyl paraben, methyl paraben,
Propellants- gases used in the food packaging industry	Argon, butane, carbon dioxide, helium, isobutene, nitrogen, nitrous oxide

Sequestrants- one type of preservatives & anti-oxidants	Poly-valent metal (copper, iron & nickel) ions, calcium chloride, oxystearin
Stabilizers - give foods a firmer texture. & stabilize emulsions.	Calcium lactobionate/gluconate, agar, pectin
Sweeteners –sugar substitutes	Sorbitol, mannitol, glycerin, aspartame, acesulfame, alitame, cyclamates, erythritol, saccharin, thaumatin
Tenderizing agents- tenderizes the tough meat and other products	Papain, bromlin, ficin, sodium tripolyphosphate (STPP)
Thickeners- increase viscosity and also act as binders	All food gums and mucilages like gum tragacanth, guar gum, locust bean gum, gelatin, pectins, carboxy methyl cellulose (CMC), poly-sorbates, algenic acid, arabino- gal-actor
Tracer gas- allows for package integrity testing to prevent foods from being exposed to atmosphere, thus guaranteeing shelf life	Carbon dioxide, helium, nitrogen

The above list does not even cover 1 % of food additives. The list is expanding at a rapid rate every year, even though the FDA and the European Food Safety Authority (EFSA) are strict in granting permission for new products and banning some of the already listed products periodically. Although the food additives got FDA or EFSA approval, many of the food chemicals are not good for health in the long run. The FDA, EFSA, NRC, ISI, BIS and other testing authorities will test the new chemicals in their laboratories, chemically, biochemically, nutritionally as well as biologically, and with laboratory animals, for few weeks or months and give the approval as safe products. It is not practical to test them in humans for decades to find their side effects.

Now all the food additives are given a code number, like E501, E385, E575 etc. Most of these so-called safe, approved food additives or chemicals are called **Generally Recognized As Safe (GRAS)**. They will exhibit their **bad** side effects **only after using them for several decades.** These bad side effects may include:

carcinogenic effect, addiction, overeating, obesity, interfering with body metabolism, destroying some natural nutrients present in the foods, immuno-suppression, habit forming, lethargy, diabetogenic, cholesterol raising, causing hypertension, allergic properties, gastro-intestinal, respiratory, CVD, neurological, psychological, hematological, musculoskeletal problems and numerous other chronic health issues.

Some of the food additives banned in USA are in use in Europe, Japan and other countries, and vice versa is also true. In case of developing countries, no such ban exists, resulting in indiscriminate use of cheap, banned, harmful food chemicals and artificial substitutes for natural products. Some of the banned chemicals are ajinomoto (MSG), MKG, BHA, BHT, caramide, coumarin, dulcin, nitrates, nitrites, propionates, bromates, nisin, natamycin, rMGH, rBST, azodic carbonamide, olestra, and many more in several hundreds.

Despite many regulations, many unsafe food additives are indiscriminately incorporated into the foods we ingest, especially in soft drinks, bakery products, further processed fruits, meats and vegetable products, resulting in emergence of several chronic health hazards, as mentioned above. Some food additives will clog up the digestive system, leading to IBS. Artificial sweeteners used as substitutes for sugar to keep the food energy (calories) low, are more dangerous than sugar by causing several health issues, including cancer. They are as dangerous as that of pesticide and herbicide residues in foods. Hence, to overcome all these health hazards, we must avoid food additives and junk foods containing these additives. We have to consume wholesome homemade foods; preferably, go back to grandma's foods.

Chapter 12

Immunity and Disease Resistance

Prevention is better than cure → but immunity is better than prevention.

Immunity is the ability of the body to overcome and withstand outbreaks of various diseases or to have better disease resistance. Immunity includes general resistance to simple non-specific diseases or conditions like fever, flu, diarrhea, headache, stomachache etc. It also includes resistance to specific diseases caused by bacterial, viral and parasitic diseases. Immunity is of different types, as follows:

- General immunity
- Specific immunity
- Active immunity
- Passive immunity
- Natural immunity

General immunity is the overall ability of a person to withstand any disease, compared to other persons. This general immunity will be partly due to the genetic makeup of the individuals and/or their better level of nutrition and environment. **Specific immunity** is the immunity for a specific contagious disease caused by virus or bacteria which occurs either due to previous exposure (infection) to the disease or vaccination against the disease. This specific immunity is for that particular disease only and not for other diseases.

Active immunity is just like specific immunity, but it includes immunity for other diseases also at a time, which may be due to multiple vaccinations and/or exposures. **Passive immunity** is a short time immunity for particular diseases, due to the administration of anti-serums (ATS), immunoglobulins, colostrum etc. **Natural immunity** is for species, genera, breed, race, who are naturally resistant to some diseases which are common in other species etc. Humans are naturally resistant to many diseases of animals and the vice versa is also true. Afro-Asians are more susceptible for CVD than Mediterranean inhabitants.

Immunity will increase the general disease resistance power and health status of the individual. Vaccination failures and breakdown of immunity are more common, due to improper vaccination, poor nutrition, mycotoxins, various kinds of stress, autoimmune diseases, pollution and many more reasons. There are several immune-suppressive diseases, which will not only cause that particular disease, but also results in general breakdown of immunity. Overall, general immunity will increase the disease resistance power of the individual, prevent disease outbreaks and thereby results in longevity of the individual. Nutritionally balanced and toxin-free natural/organic foods will boost the general immunity in individuals.

Moreover, specific nutrients, food habits and lifestyle play a major role in immunity development and disease resistance.

Role of nutrients in immunity development
All vitamins (except vitamin K), manganese, zinc, copper, selenium, sufficient balanced protein omega-3 fatty acids (α LNA, EPA and DHA) and several herbal/spices active principles in the diet, will boost immunity and disease resistance. We need about 1 g of omega-3 fatty acids, especially from fish per day. Various nutrients in the food, especially micronutrients will play a major role in immunity development, as shown in **Table-12.1**.

Besides the nutrients, certain non-nutrients like probiotics, herbs, spices, and certain specific compounds also possess immune-modulating properties. These immune-modulators in foods will boost the general immunity in individuals, prevent breakdown of immunity due to toxins and diseases, prevent vaccination failure, act as anti-stressors, tonics, toxin neutralizers, anti-viral agents and rejuvenate the immune system in the body.

Table-12-1: Role of nutrients in immunity-related functions

Nutrient	Immunity-related functions
Proteins	B-cell immunity function debilitated, atrophy of thymus, supplies essential amino acids, growth
Arginine	Augments T-cell response
Lysine	Check viral proliferation
Omega-3 fatty acids	Increase the concentration of T-cells and cytokines, increases good HDLC
Vitamin-A	WBC synthesis, invasion of macrophages to kill microbes
Vitamin-E	Natural anti-oxidant. Production of Interleukin-2, which kills microbes and cancer cells, cell integration
B-complex	RBC & WBC production, cell mediated immunity
Vitamin-C	Natural anti-oxidant. Prevents stress, anti-viral, killer cells, lymphocytes & interferon production
Manganese	Macrophage activity, enhances natural killer cells, bone density
Zinc	Immunodeficiency diseases and certain forms of cancer. Impaired thymus function, WBC production, serum IgM production, plaque forming cell response
Iron	Blastogenic response, circulating T-cells, humoral immunity antigen specific antibody titre, lactoferrin production, which invades microbes, hemoglobin synthesis
Copper	T-cell controlled infections, T-cell mitogen response, phagocytic cell anti-inflammatory effect
Selenium	Production of cytokines, prevents virus multiplication, especially influenza virus
Chromium	WBC respond to fight infection, insulin production

As stated above, these immune-modulators in foods will boost the general immunity in individuals, prevent breakdown of immunity due to toxins and diseases, prevent vaccination failure, act as anti-stressors, tonics, toxin neutralizers, anti-viral agents and rejuvenate the immune system in the body. Besides the above nutrients, several herbs and spices also have immune-modulating properties. Details of the immune-modulating and other health benefits of various herbs and spices are discussed in Chapter Thirteen, Herbs and Spices. As mentioned in Table-12-1, to boost immunity, one must consume foods rich or well balanced with the above nutrients. Moreover, they must avoid various immune-suppressors, mentioned below.

Immunity suppressors:
Unlike immunity boosters, there are also certain immunity suppressors. Several infectious and non-infectious diseases like autoimmune diseases, acquired immune deficiency syndrome (AIDS), mycotoxins, hepatitis, nephritis, spleen, bone marrow and lymph nodes infections, tuberculosis, certain types of cancers etc. causes immune suppression by destroying the T-cells, WBC, bone marrow, spleen, thymus, and lymph nodes, ultimately leading to breakdown of immunity.

Free radicals:
About 5% of oxygen used by the cells during respiration will be converted into free radicals. They are highly reactive chemicals which damage the cell membranes as well as DNA, resulting in cell death. These free radicals will specifically damage the nervous tissues and immune system. They will cause premature ageing, due to initiation and progression of many diseases, and breakdown of immunity. Antioxidants will protect the tissues from damage by the free radicals.

Antioxidants:
Antioxidants will protect the tissues from damage by the free radicals. Nutrients like vitamins A, C & E, selenium, zinc, and certain B-complex group of vitamins will act as natural antioxidants and protect the cells. Besides these nutrients, many non-nutrients active

principles present in fresh vegetables and fruits and in certain herbs, also have antioxidant properties. Carotenoid pigments, lutein, oryzanol, lycopene, nirangenin, reservetriol, coenzyme-Q10 etc. have antioxidant properties.

Many people are interested in antioxidant vitamins (A, C and E). This is due to suggestions from large observational studies comparing healthy adults consuming large amounts of these vitamins with those who didn't. However, these observations are subject to bias and don't prove a cause-and-effect relationship. **Scientific evidence does not suggest that consuming antioxidant vitamins can eliminate the need to reduce blood pressure, lower blood cholesterol or stop smoking cigarettes.** Clinical trials are underway to find out whether increased vitamin antioxidant intake may have an overall benefit. However, a recent large, placebo-controlled, randomized study failed to show any benefit from vitamin E on heart disease. Although antioxidant supplements are not recommended, antioxidant food sources—especially plant-derived foods such as fruits, vegetables, whole-grain foods and vegetable oils—are recommended.

Chapter 13

Herbs and Spices

A ll natural herbal food additives, condiments and spices we are using in our day-to-day cooking (except salt and sugar) to enhance the flavor and taste of the foods possess several medicinal, health promoting, general tonic and immune-modulating properties. These include all types of peppers, turmeric, ginger, garlic, coriander, fenugreek, mint, basil, cinnamon, cloves, cardamom, aniseeds, cumin seeds, mustard etc. They are good stomachic, digestive and carminative additives, and they promote insulin secretion and revitalize the liver and other organs. This is due to the presence of many health promoting active principles and antioxidants contained in them. Some, like turmeric, garlic etc. possess anti-viral, anti-parasitic, anti-fungal, immune-modulating, anti-microbial, and anti-carcinogenic properties. At the same time, they are safe, without any side effects.

Is spicy food good for health?
Yes, because all spices, like aniseeds, basil, caraway, cardamom, red/green/orange/yellow chili peppers, white and black peppers, celery, cinnamon, cloves, coriander, cumin seeds, curry leaves, fenugreek, dill, garlic, ginger, mint, onion, oregano, parsley, rosemary, sage, turmeric etc. have several health promoting principles (**Table-13-1**) with no side effects. Still, many people believe that chili pepper and black pepper are very hot and must be used to the minimum; otherwise, they will cause acidity, ulcers and IBS. In fact, gastric ulcers are caused by the bacteria, ***Helicobacter***

pylori or due to long-term use of nonsteroidal anti-inflammatory drugs (NSAIDs), such as aspirin and ibuprofen, but not due to eating chilies and peppers. If hot pepper is taken in an empty stomach by an ulcer patient, there will be some burning sensation, just like applying tincture of iodine on a fresh wound.

However, our dieticians are still advising us to avoid spicy foods with/without knowing their health promoting properties. **That is totally wrong advice.** It is now well established and scientifically proved that all the condiments and spices we are using in our cooking have several health promoting active principles and anti-oxidants, as mentioned in **Table-13-1**. Many herbs will help in digestion by secreting digestive enzymes. As food additives, we cannot use spices at higher levels due to their strong flavor and taste. Hence, the question of using them at higher levels does not arise.

Among the spices and condiments we are using regularly, garlic, turmeric, onion, black pepper, chili (red) pepper, ginger, mustard, basil, oregano, dill, rosemary, *ajwan* (caraway), fenugreek, curry leaves, coriander, mint, cinnamon, cardamom, cloves, cumin seeds, and many more possess immune boosting, anti-oxidant and health promoting properties. They also act as correctives; they will correct minor imbalances in food, digestive problems and act as a general tonic. Based on these authenticated data on the health promoting properties of herbs and spices, many of them are not only plentiful in grocery stores and supermarkets, but are also available in pharmacies as health supplements for many chronic diseases like arthritis, cancer, CVD, diabetes, hypertension, neurological problems, obesity etc. in the USA, Canada, China, Europe Japan and many other countries.

Use of herbs in ancient medicine:
Herbs have been used as medicine throughout the history by all cultures and for numerous illnesses. Archaeologists, examining remains of a Neanderthal burial site called Shanidar IV in Iraq and in the Mohenjo-Daro and Harappa in the Indus valley, have found evidence that humans used herbs some 60,000 years B.C. Over

5,000 years B.C., the ancient Sumerians in Mesopotamia started keeping written records of herbs and their medicinal purposes. The Chinese began using herbal medicines in their traditional medicine some 5,000 years B.C., followed by the ancient Egyptians 1,500 years B.C., who expanded the use of herbs and spices such as garlic. In Europe, herbs were used extensively by the Greeks starting in 300 A.D. In America, Native Americans such as the Cherokee, Catawba and Hopi tribes have used herbs and teas such as blue cohosh, partridgeberry and licorice for thousands of years to treat disease. Flowers, leaves, berries, roots and stems—they all go into the herbal mix to prevent and treat health conditions like high blood pressure. Also, many ancient herbal properties have been captured so they can be used synthetically today in large amounts. Much of the conventional medicine we take today was developed from herbs. The World Health Organization estimates that 4 billion people (that's about 60% of the people on earth) use herbal medicine for some aspect of their primary health care.

The first authenticated herbal system of medicine, called as **Ayurveda**, was developed in ancient India some 5,000 years ago and is still followed in India and many other countries. Another herbal system of medicine, **Siddha,** is being followed now in South India. The **Unani** system of medicine, mostly followed by Southeast Asian Muslims, also uses herbs and spices. Several medical colleges in India are now offering graduate, post-graduate and research degrees in **Ayurveda, Siddha and Unani** systems of medicines. The Chinese system of medicine is also using mostly herbal medicines. Even in present day modern medicine several herbal extracts or active principles are used as medicines and diet plays a major role in speedy recovery of the patients from ailments. If you visit the supermarkets and pharmacies in the USA, Canada, Japan, Europe and China, you will find herbal medicines from all over the world. Many individuals are using these safe, non-prescription herbal medicines for prevention and control of chronic diseases like CVD, diabetes, obesity, hypertension, cholesterol control, neurological problems, musculoskeletal and gastrointestinal disorders.

Table-13.1: Active principles and functions of commonly used herbs and spices

Name of the herb/spice	Active principles	Functions
Garlic	Allicin, allelic sulfide, aojene	Anti-microbial, anti-viral, natural antibiotic, reduces cholesterol, CVD, BP & TGL
Curry leaves (*Murraya koenigi*)	Koenigin, murrayin	Stomachic, general tonic, antioxidant, anti-diabetic, reduces cholesterol, BP & TGL
Coriander seeds & leaves (cilantro)	Borneol, cineole, linoleic acid, linalool,	Stomachic, controls liver disorders, diarrhea, reduces BP, arthritis & increases milk secretion
Cornelian cherry (*Cornus mas*)	Anthocyanins, pelargonin, cyanidin	Reduces cholesterol & CVD, antioxidant, anti-inflammatory
Mint	Peppermint oil, flavonoids	Antioxidant, ---do---
Ginger	gingerolin	Reduces cholesterol, BP and sugar, anti-diabetic
Onion	Quercetin & biflavanoids	Anti-inflammatory, anti-cancer, anti-microbial, lowers blood sugar, cholesterol, BP & heat stroke
Fenugreek seeds,	Methyl- hydroxyl- chalcone- polymer (MHCP)	Stomachic, reduces cholesterol and sugar, anti-diabetic
Cardamom	Flavonoids, anti-oxidants	Reduces cholesterol, BP and sugar, anti-diabetic
Cloves	---do---	--do--
Cinnamon	Cinnamaldehyde	---do--
Turmeric	Curcumin & curcuminoid group of flavonoids	Anti-carcinogenic, anti-oxidant, anti-viral, anti-bacterial, anti-parasitic, anti-fungal, anti-protozoan, immune-modulator, anti-inflammatory, reduces all respiratory diseases, improves vision by improving retinal pigmentation, rods & cones.
Red, green, orange, yellow pepper, chilies,	Capsanthin, carotenoid pigments, especially lutein, flavonoid compounds	Eye (retina) tonic, act synergistically with turmeric and marigold petals in improving vision, prevents night blindness, MD, RP, cataract & other eye diseases. Reduces cholesterol, reduces blood sugar

Black pepper	Pepperolin, flavonoids	Reduces cholesterol & BP. Act synergistically with turmeric & boosts the action of turmeric.
Piper longum	piperin	Liver tonic, prevents lipid peroxidation
Oregano	Carvacrol, antioxidants	Boost immunity, anti-parasitic
Thyme	Flavonoids	Boost immunity, antibacterial
Rosemary	Flavonoids, carnosic acid	Eye tonic, anti-stress, anti-inflammatory
Watermelon	Cucurbocitrin	Dilates blood vessels & reduces BP
Grapes (red & black)	Resveratrol, flavonoids	Lowers cholesterol & BP
Waterlily & lotus- roots & tuber	Nymphin, nowchalin	Reduce blood sugar, controls diabetes and obesity
Guava fruit & leaves	Nerolidiol, sitostreol, leucocyanidin, caryophyllene, b-bisabolene, p-selinene	Antioxidant, anti-inflammatory, reduces LDLC & sugar, controls obesity & diarrhea
Avocado	Flavonoids, anti-oxidants	Reduces BP & cholesterol
Oranges & limes	---do--- , vit.-C	Immunity booster, anti-cancer
Beetroot	--do---	Reduces BP & cholesterol
Mushrooms	Muscarin, flavonoids	----do---
Embilica officinalis, Indian gooseberry, amla	Anti-oxidants, flavonoids	Liver tonic, anti-cancer, immune booster, rejuvenator, anti-stress
Basil, Thulasi (holy basil) & white basil	Eugenol, eugenic acid, carvecrol	Immunomodulation, reduces cholesterol & BP, anti-microbial
Flax seeds, canola, chia, fish oil	n-3 FA- Alpha-linoleic acid(LNA), EPA, DHA	Lowers risk of cardio-vascular diseases, Reduces bad cholesterol
Phyllanthus neruri (ground amla)	Phyllanthin, ascorbic acid, emblicanin, hypophyllanthin,	Rejuvenates liver cells, cures all types of jaundice, detoxification

Andrographis paniculata	Andrographolide	Rejuvenates hepatic cells, anti-viral, anti-oxidant
Solanum nigram (black night shade)	Solanin	Stomachic, cardiac tonic, appetizer, prevents gastric ulcers & cancer
Anisochilus carmorus-karpooravalli	Anisochilin (thick leaved, strong tasting lavender)	Control cough, sour throat, cold and wheezing
Tribulus terrestris, palleru, small herb, with thorny fruits	Antioxidants	Diuretic, tonic
Grape seed & pulp	Resveratrol, lycopene, nirangenin	Anti-oxidant, increases good HDL cholesterol
Citrus pulp, tea waste	Flavonoid compounds	Anti-oxidant, anti-cancer
Various berries, including gooseberry, blueberry	Anthocyanins & many other antioxidants	Powerful anti-oxidants, anti-cancer, liver tonic
Cranberry, prunes	Flavonoids	Diuretic, prevents kidney stones
Broccoli, cauliflower, cabbage & turnip	Sulforaphane & many other antioxidants	Anti-cancer, antioxidant
Soy, clover	Isoflavonoids & many other antioxidants	Prevents arterial/capillary blocking
Spirulina, azolla	LNA, xanthophylls, chlorophyll	Yolk pigments, reduces cholesterol & stress, anti-oxidant, eye tonic
Neem – *Azadirachta indica*	Numbin, numbidin	Anti-microbial, anti-mold, anti-fungal, controls sugar and BP,
Glycyrrhiza glabra	Licorice	Anti-microbial, stomachic
Azaracta caryophyllus	Azaractin	Increase T-cell immunity
Alfalfa	Sataivin	Immune-modulator
Andrographis paniculata	Andrographolide	Prevents liver damage, neutralizes toxins & pesticides, immunomodulation, rejuvenator of vital organs

Picroriza kurroa	Picroliv	Immunomodulation, rejuvenator
Tinosporin	Antioxidants	Stimulates immunity,
Withania sominifera: Aswagandha)	Isopelletierine, anaferine, withanolides	Immunomodulation, rejuvenator
Ginseng (Ginseng panax)	Ginsenosides	Rejuvenator, adaptogen
Terminalia chebula	Lupeol, friedelin, glucopanoside	Immunomodulation, rejuvenator, anti-fungal
Trichopus zeylanicum (Arogya pacha)	Punigluconin, flavonoids	Anti-stress, cures AIDS, immune-modulator, rejuvenator
Tinospora cardifolia	Tinosporin	Stimulates humoral & cell mediated immunity
Graviola /soursop/ guyabano fruit	Graviolin	Powerful anti-cancer agent, & immune-modulator
Cassia augustifolia (swarna patri)	Emodins, chrysophanic acid	Anti-microbial, blood purifier
Bringaraj / Asteraceae *Eclypta alba*	Wedelolactone, furanocoumarins, oleanane & taraxastan	Liver cell rejuvenator, toxin neutralizer, immunomodulation,
Nothapodyte s foetida	Camptothecin	Approved anti-cancer drug
Indian sarasaparilla, *Nalleru, Parandai,*	*Cissus quadrangularis*	Galactogogue, reduces fever, syphilis, blood purifier
Green tea (without sugar & milk)	Theoflavin, theobromin, coffin, catechin	Weight reduction, sugar control, cholesterol reduction
Rice bran oil (see lipids chapter)	Gama oryzanol & many other antioxidants	Powerful anti-oxidant, controls cholesterol & sugar
Garcinia cambogia	Hydroxyl- citric acid	Suppresses appetite, melts body fat & eliminate it. Suitable for weight loss
Cassia augustifolia (Swarna	Chrysophanic acid, aloe-emodins,	Blood purifier, correct stomach disorders, anti-microbial, laxative

pathri –Nela-thangedu)	tinnelvellin, glycosides	
Nothapodytes foetida	Camptothecin	Herbal anti-cancer drug- on sale in USA
Clitoria ternatea (conch flower climber)	Clitorin	Diuretic, cathartic, laxative
Cardiospermum helicacaban	Cardiospermin-present in all parts of this creeper	Rheumatism, nervous disorders, laxative, skin tonic

Besides condiments and spices, several vegetables and fruits, medicinal herbs like Ginseng (*Panax ginseng*), Aswagandha (*Withania sominifera*), basil, holy basil/Thulasi (*Ocimum sanctum*), white basil (*Ocimum album*), *Phyllanthus neruri*, *Andrographis paniculata*, *Solanum nigram* (*black night shade*), alfalfa, *Andrographis paniculata*, *Picroriza kurroa*, *Embilica officinalis* (Amla/Indian goose berry), *Eclypta alba* and many more possess anti-bacterial, anti-viral, carminative, stomachic, stimulant, immune-modulator and powerful antioxidant properties, as mentioned in Table-13-1.

- Mustard/canola/rapeseeds are rich in Ω-3 fatty acids, similar to fish, walnuts, flax and chia seeds. This oil will increase good cholesterol- HDLC.

- Fenugreek seeds and leaves are rich sources of organic chromium, present in insulin. Hence, it increases insulin secretion, so it is good for diabetic and pre-diabetics.

- Gurmar (chakkara kolli- sugar killer), banana leaf, flower and stem extract, bitter gourd, avocados, custard apple seeds, Indian *naga* fruit seeds are very good to control diabetes. Hence, they are used in herbal medicines preparation for diabetes.

- *Phyllanthus neruri, Eclypta alba* and Indian gooseberry are good for liver and cures all liver diseases, jaundice and hepatitis of all forms.

- All fruits and vegetables are rich in potassium, which is good for the heart and reduces blood pressure. They are also rich in anti-oxidants and immune-modulators. **Always use garden fresh vegetables and fruits**. Their health promoting properties will diminish with storage, processing, cooking and further processing. Even peeling of skin and removing of seeds in certain fruits and vegetables will remove valuable nutrients, active principles and fiber.

- Most of the spices like garlic, turmeric, onion, ginger are anti-microbial. Hence, they are safe and good substitutes for antibiotics. Turmeric powder contains curcumin, which is antiviral, antimicrobial and prevents cancer, especially breast cancer.

- Graviola or sour-sop fruit (native of Brazil), custard apple, *Rama phal*, belonging to the same family, are good anti-cancer agents. They have 'Graviolin', a powerful anti-cancer active principle, used for cancer treatment in many countries. Many pharmaceutical companies have made futile attempts to synthesize and patent this Graviolin.

- *Garcinia cambogia* fruits contain hydroxylcitric acid. It suppresses appetite, melts body fat and eliminates it. Therefore, it is an ideal fruit for weight loss and obesity control.

Guava, papaya, pineapple, grape, kiwi, strawberry, raspberry, custard apple and minor less known fruits and berries like *Badri (Zuzupus, regu, Ilandai), Indian naga* fruit and wood apple, are fruits superior to regular fruits like banana and apple. These fruits have several active principles, like anthocyanin, nirangin, resveratrol, lycopene, flavonoids, embicanin, murrayin and many more health promoting **anti-oxidant** principles, with high **FRAP (Ferric Reduction Anti-Oxidant Power)** value. Fruits are now ranked based on their FRAP values. As such guava, wood apple, Indian *naga and* zizipus fruits, blueberries, blackberries, grapes, pineapple, kiwi, raspberries and strawberries are top 10 ranking fruits, based on their **FRAP** values. On the other hand, the most common fruits, bananas and apples, rank lower. However, all fresh fruits are good for health.

Foods, vegetables, spices and herbs **good for the heart and to reduce BP, bad cholesterol and sugar** are garlic, onion, ginger, cinnamon, cardamom, curry leaves, fish oil, flax, chia, red grapes, beetroot (not sugar beet), carrot, soy protein, mushrooms, bitter guard, cucumber, mint, coriander, red capsicum, watermelon and herbs like, *Withania sominifera (Aswagandha), Terminalia chebula), Ginseng (Ginseng panax), gymnema sylvestre* (sugar killer, chakkera kolli, gurmar), *and Trichopus zeylanicum (Arogya pacha),*

Garlic - Garlic contains allicin, a substance which has antibacterial, antioxidant, lipid-lowering and anti-hypertension properties, by dilating the blood vessels. In a pilot study made at Clinical Research Center of New Orleans on whether garlic could lower blood pressure, nine patients with severe hypertension were given a garlic preparation containing 1.3 % allicin. Sitting blood pressure fell with a significant decrease in diastolic blood pressure only five to 14 hours after the dose. Moreover, it was proven in a 2009 study that fresh garlic has more potent cardio-protective properties than processed garlic.

Cinnamon - Cinnamon is another tasty seasoning that requires little effort to include in your daily diet, and it may bring your blood pressure numbers down. Consuming cinnamon every day has been shown to lower blood pressure in people with diabetes. Include more cinnamon in your diet by sprinkling it on your breakfast cereal, oatmeal, and even in your coffee. At dinner, cinnamon enhances the flavor of stir-fries, curries, and stews. Cinnamon not only prevents heart disease, it can also prevent diabetes.

The Center for Applied Health Sciences in Ohio conducted a study of 22 subjects, half of which were given 250 mg of water-soluble cinnamon daily, while the other half were given placebo. It was discovered that those who drank cinnamon had a 13 to 23 percent increase in antioxidants connected with lowering blood sugar levels. As stated above, cinnamon is another tasty seasoning that requires little effort to include in your daily diet and that may bring your blood pressure numbers down. Cinnamon combined with magnesium and lifestyle changes may lead to overall reductions in blood pressure up to 25 mm Hg.

Onions - Onions contain quercetin, an antioxidant flavonol found to prevent heart disease and stroke. In a research study published in the *Journal of Nutrition*, subjects with hypertension experienced a decrease in their blood pressure by 7 mm Hg systolic and 5 mm Hg diastolic as opposed to those who were taking placebo.

Olives - This herb is a significant part of the Mediterranean diet, recognized to be one of the healthiest in the world. Oil made from olives has been found to reduce blood pressure. In a study conducted on the importance of olive oil, Dr. L. Aldo Ferrara, Associate Professor at the *Frederico II University of Naples* in Italy discovered that the daily use of 40 grams of olive oil reduced the dosage of blood pressure medication in hypertensive patients by about 50 percent. Polyphenols in extra-virgin olive oil was credited for the significant reduction of blood pressure.

Oregano - This herb contains the compound carvacrol, which has been proven to be effective against high blood pressure. In a study conducted on animal subjects by researchers from *Eskisehir Osmangazi University* in Turkey, carvacrol was found to reduce heart rate, mean arterial pressure as well as the systolic and diastolic blood pressures.

Hibiscus - Hibiscus tea (from the plant *Hibiscus sabdariffa*) and supplements have been found to lower blood pressure in human studies. A systematic review of four randomized controlled trials found that in two studies testing the effects of hibiscus tea to black tea, hibiscus tea was associated with reduced systolic and diastolic blood pressure. Two studies comparing hibiscus extract to angiotensin converting enzyme (ACE) inhibitors (captopril or lisinopril) also showed reductions for hibiscus tea groups, but the effects were generally less than those of the ACE-inhibitor groups.

Cat's claw - Cat's claw is an herbal medicine used in traditional Chinese practice to treat hypertension, as well as neurological health problems. Studies of cat's claw as a treatment for hypertension indicate that it may be helpful in reducing blood pressure by acting on calcium channels in your cells. It also contains an anti-inflammatory agent that blocks the production of the hormone prostaglandin, which contributes to inflammation and pain. You can find cat's claw in supplement form at many health food stores, but it is also widely available as a tea.

Hawthorn - This herb has been traditionally used to treat high blood pressure. In one study conducted in Reading, UK, 79 type-2 diabetic patients were randomized to receive 1200 mg of hawthorn extract, while another group received medication for high blood pressure. Results revealed that patients taking hawthorn by the end of the 16th week showed a reduction in their mean diastolic pressure. Hawthorn is an herbal remedy for high blood pressure that has been used in traditional Chinese medicine for thousands of years. Decoctions of hawthorn seem to have a whole host of benefits on cardiovascular health, including reduction of blood pressure, the prevention of clot formation, and an increase in blood circulation. You can take hawthorn as a pill, a liquid extract, or a tea.

Cardamom - In one study published in the *Indian Journal of Biochemistry and Biophysics*, 20 subjects newly diagnosed with primary hypertension were administered 3 g of cardamom powder. After the end of the three months, all the subjects experienced feelings of well-being without any side effects. Moreover, the study was able to demonstrate that blood pressure was effectively reduced. It also improved antioxidant status while breaking down blood clots without significantly altering blood lipids and fibrinogen levels. Cardamom is a seasoning that comes from India, and is often used in the foods of South Asia. A study investigating the health effects of cardamom found that participants given powdered cardamom daily for several months saw significant reductions in their blood pressure readings. You can include cardamom seeds or the powder in spice rubs, in soups and stews, and even in baked goods for a special flavor and a positive health benefit. As with many spices, cardamom has been demonstrated to have antioxidant properties. Kikuzaki, Kawai, and Nakatani (2001) examined extracts from black cardamom (*Amomum subulatum*) for their ability to scavenge radicals. A study investigating the health effects of cardamom found that participants given powdered cardamom daily for several months saw significant reductions in their blood pressure readings.

Basil - Basil is a delicious herb that goes well in a variety of foods. It also might help lower your blood pressure. Extract of basil has been shown to lower blood pressure, although only briefly. Adding fresh basil to your diet is easy and certainly can't hurt. Keep a small pot of the herb in your kitchen garden and add the fresh leaves to pastas, soups, salads, and casseroles. Basil is originally native to Iran, India, and other tropical regions of Asia, but now it is widely available throughout the world. Basil has antioxidant, antimutagenic, anticarcinogenic, antiviral, and antibacterial properties. It also helps lower your blood pressure. Extract of basil has been shown to lower blood pressure.

Ginger - Ginger may help control blood pressure, as it has been shown to improve blood circulation and relax the muscles surrounding blood vessels. Commonly used in Asian foods, ginger is a very versatile ingredient that can also be used in sweets or beverages. Chop, mince, or grate fresh ginger into stir-fries, soups, and noodle or vegetable dishes, or add it to desserts or tea for a refreshing taste.

Coriander seeds and leaves (cilantro) - The active principles in it are borneol, cineole, and linalool. They control diarrhea, arthritis, liver disorders and hypertension. It is a good stomachic and liver tonic. It also increases milk secretion.

Turmeric - It is a wonder spice from India and is now spread throughout the world. It is not only used as a spice, but as a medicine throughout the world. Its active principle, **curcumin,** is available as capsules in all super markets and pharmacies in many developed countries. Turmeric is antimicrobial and accepted as a natural food antibiotic, along with garlic. It is anti-inflammatory, anti-oxidant, reduces CVD, hypertension, Alzheimer's, cholesterol, several types of cancer, heals ulcers, wounds, and controls indigestion, bloating and gas.

Hence, even in western countries, where there is no herbal/Ayurveda system of medicine in vogue, several spices and herbal preparations are available in all pharmacies and supermarkets in the form of capsules/powders as natural food supplements which can be taken as preventive medicine for control of several chronic diseases without any prescription, because they are safe. There are no curative medicines for many chronic diseases in the modern allopathic system. These medicines are mostly symptoms suppressants and not disease curatives. Moreover, they have several adverse side effects. Some of them are synthetic replica of the herbal active principles. So, very soon herbal/Ayurveda system of medicine will be introduced in the developed western countries.

Chapter 14

Genetically Modified Foods

According to the WHO, "Genetically modified organisms (GMOs)" can be defined as organisms (i.e. plants, animals or microorganisms) in which the genetic material (DNA) has been altered in a way that does not occur naturally by mating and/or natural recombination. The foods produced from, or using GM organisms, are often referred to as **GM foods.** In the USA, the USDA and FDA favor the use of the term, "genetic engineering" over "genetic modification" as the more precise term.

After World War II, when the "**green revolution**" started, several "**hybrid crops**" were introduced in order to increase the crop yield to feed the entire world. At that time there was resistance from some traditional people and NGOs against hybrid crops. If those hybrid crops were not introduced at that time, half the world might have died due to starvation. Such resistance was noticed for GM crops also when it was introduced around 1993. With ever-growing global population, combined with reduced availability of cultivable land, **agriculture scientists have concluded that there is no alternative to GM foods to avoid starvation deaths in the world**. Plants that are genetically engineered (GE), or modified, have been selectively bred and enhanced with genes to withstand common problems faced by the farmers, like crop failure due to drought, pests, low yield and many emerging diseases.

History of GM crops

The GM crops have been in use for more than two decades, but the research was started in the early 1980s. China was the first country to commercialize a transgenic crop in 1993, with the introduction of virus-resistant tobacco. The first GM food approved for release was the Flavr Savr tomato in 1994, developed by Calgene. It was engineered to have a longer shelf life by inserting an antisense gene that delayed ripening. In 1995, *Bacillus thuringiensis* (Bt) potato was approved for cultivation, making it the first biological-pesticide producing crop to be approved in the USA. Later, several genetically modified crops like, canola, corn, cotton, soybeans, squash, sugar beet, zucchini, papaya, pineapple, tangerines, wheat, rice etc. were produced. Genetically modified crops are mainly developed with the intention of improving their disease resistance and their yield.

By 2010, 29 countries had planted commercialized biotech crops and a further 31 countries had granted regulatory approval for transgenic crops to be imported. USA was the leading country in the production of GM foods in 2011, with twenty-five GM crops having received regulatory approval. In 2015, 92% of corn, 94% of soybeans, and 94% of cotton produced in the US were genetically modified strains.

The first genetically modified animal to be approved for food use was **Aqua-Advantage Salmon** in 2015. The salmon were transformed with a growth hormone-regulating gene from a Pacific Chinook salmon and a promoter from an ocean pout, enabling it to grow year-round instead of only during spring and summer.

In April 2016, a **white button mushroom** (*Agaricus bisporus*), modified by using the CRISPR technique, received *de facto* approval in the United States by USDA. According to the USDA, the number of field releases for genetically engineered organisms has grown from four in 1985 to an average of about 800 per year. Cumulatively, more than 17,000 releases had been approved through September 2013, and the cumulative approval of genetically engineered organisms up to 2016 has crossed 20,000 releases.

Now scientists are focusing on **bio-fortification of crops** to produce crops fortified with extra nutrients; in addition, to produce higher yields from the same planted area. With the creation of **golden rice** in 2000, scientists had genetically modified food to increase its nutrient value for the first time. This variety of rice has more carotenoid pigments, a precursor of vitamin-A, which will prevent blindness. Further research on this aspect has resulted in the development of cassava (tapioca/mandioca), corn, canola, soya, sugar beet, papaya, pineapple, tangerine etc., bio-fortified with additional nutrients so that people will not suffer from common nutrient deficiency diseases. GM crops have the potential to strengthen farming and food security by granting more certainty against the unpredictable factors of nature. These resistances and higher yields hold great promise for the developing world and for global food security.

GM crops controversies
Genetically modified food controversies are disputes over the use of foods and other goods derived from genetically modified crops and other uses of genetic engineering in food production. The dispute involves consumers, farmers, biotechnology companies, governmental regulators, non-governmental organizations, and scientists. The key areas of controversy related to genetically modified food are whether such food should be labeled, the role of government regulators, the objectivity of scientific research and publication, the effect of genetically modified crops on health and the environment, the effect on pesticide resistance, the impact of such crops for farmers, and the role of the crops in feeding the world population. In addition, products derived from GMO organisms play a role in the production of ethanol fuels and pharmaceuticals.

There is a scientific consensus that currently available food derived from GM crops poses no greater risk to human health than conventional food, but that each GM food needs to be tested on a case-by-case basis before introduction. Nonetheless, members of the public are much less likely than scientists to perceive GM foods as safe.

Specific concerns include mixing of genetically modified and non-genetically modified products in the food supply, effects of GMOs on the environment, the rigor of the regulatory process and consolidation of control of the food supply in companies that make and sell GMOs. Advocacy groups such as the Center for Food Safety, Organic Consumers Association, Union of Concerned Scientists and Greenpeace, say risks have not been adequately identified and managed, and they have questioned the objectivity of regulatory authorities.

Advantages of GM crops

1. GM crops are more environment friendly because:

- GM technology reduced the use of pesticide and other crop protection chemicals by about 10%.

- Genetically modified crops require less plowing and chemical usage.

- GM technology reduces the use of fossil fuel and CO_2 emissions. Genetic engineering can therefore help to ameliorate the effects of agriculture on the environment.

- In recent years, farming accounted for 24% of global greenhouse gas emissions and 70% of fresh water use. These two can be reduced significantly in GM crop production.

- In order to feed a world population that is expected to cross 9 billion before 2050, we need to roughly **double the crop production, using less than the present amount of land** (because some land will be used for housing and industry, and some land will be unfit for cultivation). Such doubling of crop production is almost impossible with the existing conventional/hybrid crops. Hence, GM crops that do not harm the environment are needed to achieve this goal.

- GM crops allow for greater use of no-till cultivation, which helps with carbon sequestration, soil erosion prevention and better soil fertility.

2. GM crops are more farmers' friendly because:

- Genetically modified crops are more efficient in reducing the agricultural inputs to produce more amount of food.

- Genetic modification can protect crops against threats to strong yields, such as diseases, drought, pests, and herbicides used to control weeds, and therefore, improve the efficiency of food production.

- Cultivation of Bt corn, canola, cotton, golden rice, papaya, pineapple, soya, squash, etc. led to more yields, resulting in lesser cost of production and more income to the farmers.

- Scientists are now developing GM crops that are resistant to flood, drought, and cold, which will improve agricultural resistance to climate change.

- Genetic modification helps to eliminate some of the problems faced by smallholder farmers, such as droughts, pests, and crop diseases. From 1996-2013, genetic modification added $116.9 billion to the agricultural sector, and more than 50% went to farmers in developing countries.

- Genetic modification prevents crop loss due to disease, insects, and herbicides used to control weeds, resulting in more efficient production and potentially lower food prices. According to the World Bank, agricultural sector growth is the most effective pathway for reducing poverty and increasing food access. Genetically modified crops increase farmers' revenue by reducing some input costs, including for pesticides and water, reducing crop losses, and allowing farmers more time to pursue other activities.

- GM crops also reduce insurance costs for farmers by producing more consistent yields, with reduced crop damage by pests.

- Genetic engineering research has focused on overcoming problems that affect productivity, such as disease, weeds, and pests. When crops can avoid diseases, weeds, and pests, crop yield is enhanced. When the genetic modification tool is combined with improved farm management practices, agricultural chemicals, farm machinery etc. they will act **synergistically,** resulting in still higher yields and lesser environmental pollution.

3. GM crops are more concerned with human health and food security because:

- In the past 15 years more than 2,000 studies have showed no human or environmental dangers from genetically engineered crops, with a study concluding that the **scientific research conducted so far has not detected any significant hazard directly connected with the use of GM crops.**

- The **European Commission** released a meta-analysis of 50 research projects and found that the use of biotechnology and of GE plants *per se* does not imply higher risks than does classical breeding methods or production technologies.

- Genetic modification can **improve the nutritional profile of foods**, and therefore serves as a key element in reducing global rates of malnutrition. For instance, **GM golden rice** is enhanced with **beta-carotene**, a precursor of vitamin A, a nutrient lacking in many diets around the third-world countries. So golden rice is a crucial initiative in reducing malnutrition.

- Cultivation of Bt corn, canola, cotton, golden rice, papaya, pineapple, soya, squash, etc. led to more yields and higher nutrients due to bio-fortification, resulting in lesser cost of production and more income to the farmers, and increased consumption of more nutritious foods—including fruits, vegetables and animal products—to the consumers.

Level of acceptance of GM crops:

The following statistics tell the story of the level of acceptance and use of GM crops and seeds by large and small farmers, in both the developed and developing countries. According to the independent International Service for the Acquisition of Agri-biotech Applications (ISAAA), a non-profit organization, the global area of biotech crops for 2012 was 170.3 million hectares, grown by 17.3 million farmers in 28 countries, with an average annual growth in areas cultivated of approximately 6%. More than 90% of farmers growing biotech GM crops are resource-poor farmers in developing countries. Now 60-70 percent of the foods in the United States market have some GM food ingredients.

In 2013, over 16 million smallholder farmers in developing countries grew biotech crops. Fifteen million smallholder farmers in Burkina Faso, China, India, Pakistan, and a few other developing countries grow Bt cotton. In countries with weak or non-existent extension services, farmers can face challenges in accessing GM seeds and in learning best growing techniques. Some countries ban the import of seeds, while others exclude GM seeds.

GM foods are also "natural" foods:

There is actually no FDA regulation or specific definition of the term "natural" on food labels, so there is little merit to any label claiming that a food product is natural. Typically, though, the term indicates that a food product is not highly processed and/or does not contain added colors or preservatives. Therefore, under this definition, the GM crops are not unnatural, but are natural. There is a scientific consensus that currently available foods derived from GM crops pose no greater risk to human health than conventional food, but that each GM food needs to be tested on a case-by-case basis before introduction. Since GM foods are environment, farmers and consumers friendly, as stated above, and the advocacy groups such as the Center for Food Safety, Organic Consumers Association, Union of Concerned Scientists and Greenpeace, say risks have not been adequately identified and managed, GM foods are safe and can also be used for organic food production.

Safety and legal issues:

The safety assessment of genetically engineered food products by regulatory bodies starts with an evaluation of whether or not the food is substantially equivalent to non-genetically engineered counter-parts that are already deemed fit for human consumption. No reports of ill effects have been documented in the human population from genetically modified food. There is a scientific consensus that currently available food derived from GM crops poses no greater risk to human health than conventional food, but that each GM food needs to be tested on a case-by-case basis before introduction. Nonetheless, members of the public are much less likely than scientists to perceive GM foods as safe. The legal and regulatory status of GM foods varies from country to country, with some nations banning or restricting them, and others permitting them with widely differing degrees of regulation.

Whatever may be the present status of the genetically modified crops, in the future we have to depend on them to feed the ever-growing global population, since the present crops' yield will diminish gradually, due to emerging diseases of crops and diminishing cultivable land holdings. In the meanwhile, further research will remove the myths and fears about accepting them as safe foods. Now in USA, 60-70% of the foods in the market have some GM food ingredients, which will increase further due to no ban by the regulatory authorities, the USDA and FDA. In some countries, the use of GM foods is still at a low phase at present, which will also increase gradually because of higher cost and lesser availability of non-GM foods in future.

Chapter 15

Organic Foods

Organic food production follows the principles of **Vedas** (pre-historic four Indian holy-scientific books), which say "**Live in partnership with, rather than exploit nature.**" Organic food production is more or less similar to the agricultural practices followed by our ancestors in 19th century or earlier. The quality of the food produced at that time is better than the so-called organic foods produced at present. During those days, there were no hybrid varieties, genetically modified crops, pesticides, herbicides, synthetic fertilizers like urea, NPK, DAP, and other chemicals used at present in agriculture production. The soil was fertile, not polluted with pests and other chemicals. The water used for irrigation was mostly from rivers, ponds and lakes, which were not polluted. So the crops produced during olden days were 100% organic.

Now the global scenario has entirely changed, mainly due to exploitation by humans. The population has multiplied greatly since the 19th century. At the same time, the cultivable land size has diminished due to industrialization and urbanization, and many lands are now unfit for organic crop production. Therefore, the farmers are forced to produce four to five times more crops (to feed more mouths, due to the ever-growing population) with lesser land holdings. Furthermore, many new pests and diseases of crops have emerged, damaging the crops. The soil fertility level has diminished. Therefore, agriculture scientists, under green revolution, have had to develop high yielding and more disease resistant crops, GM crops, artificial fertilizers, pesticides, herbicides and other techniques, in order to increase the crop yield to feed all the humans and animals on earth and prevent starvation deaths.

The organic crop production has to be carried out in organic certified soils only, under the strict supervision and guidance of the certifying agency, like USDA and other certifying authorities in the respective countries. The farmer cannot use artificial fertilizers, pesticides, herbicides, and other chemicals, resulting in higher cost of production and far lesser yields. If the entire world is under organic food production, the yield would not be sufficient to feed even 25% of the world population, leading to starvation deaths worldwide. To overcome this shortage to some extent, the high yielding, pest resistant and bio-fortified GM crops must be allowed worldwide for organic food production, because GM crops will be more suitable for organic food production than conventional crops, due to more disease resistance and lesser need of fertilizers. Hence, the cost of production of organic foods will be lower if GM foods are used. Moreover, regulatory authorities like USDA and FDA have accepted GM foods as natural foods and safe to consume.

Nutritionally, both organic and regular foods are equal, but regular foods may have pesticide/herbicide residues. Therefore, they have to be washed thoroughly before cooking or consumption. Even though organic foods are safe to consumers, their present market prices are 100-300% higher due to higher cost of production and lower yield. At present prices it is expensive to purchase them, and only a few people can afford them. Moreover, if the entire world produced only organic foods, the production will not be sufficient to feed the population. But those who cannot afford to purchase organic foods need not be worried. Since both non-organic and organic foods are nutritionally comparable, we can consume regular non-organic foods after thoroughly washing them under running water, or soaking them in water for few minutes, followed by rinsing, to remove pesticide residues, if any. Thereafter, they can be used safely for cooking and eating, just like any organic foods.

Organic foods cannot cater to the needs of the entire world population due to lesser availability of land for organic foods cultivation and lesser yield of organic crops. Their yields can be increased and the cost of production can be decreased if GM seeds are used for their production, which is now under consideration.

Keep the soil in good cultivable condition, with high fertility rate, by following healthy soil management and agronomy practices so that the land can be used for cultivation as long as the human race exists on earth. Improve the soil fertility by using farmyard manure collected from various animal farms and different oil cakes/meals available locally. Fallen leaves may be composted or spread over the land during the fall, so that the winter snow will accumulate over the leaves, and they will decompose and become a good manure by spring and will enrich the soil. These rotting leaves will encourage earthworms to grow, and they will aerate the soil. Take the advice of an agronomist or horticulturist to learn and implement the latest techniques in cultivation in order to increase the crop yield and protect them from pests in an organic way. Use good quality certified seeds from a reliable source. Save the land to keep the world free from starvation.

Chapter 16

Obesity and Weight Management

Any weight gain in men over 25 years of age and women over 20 years of age (except during pregnancy and lactation) is nothing but body fat deposition. For healthy living, maintain the same healthy body weight (except during pregnancy and lactation), with BMI ranging from 20 to 24, throughout your life. So check your body weight at least once a month and calculate your BMI, using the following formula. If there is any gain in your body weight and BMI, reduce your food and/or calorie intake or burn excess fat by doing extra exercise. People with BMI of above 25, especially >30 will have higher risk for CVD, diabetes, arthritis, cancer and other chronic diseases. Hence, it is advisable to maintain BMI between 20 to 24 by restricting calories and doing exercise regularly.

How to calculate your Body Mass Index (BMI)?

- BMI is an indication of body weight in relation to the height of the individual. It is calculated using this formula:

- BMI = Body weight in kg ÷ height in meters ^{2}.

- You can also calculate BMI using another formula:

- BMI = Body weight in lbs. ÷ height in inches ^{2} X 705.

- For example, if a person weighs 70 kg/154 lbs., with a height of 1.75 meters/68.9 inches, his BMI will be 70 ÷ 1.75^2 = 22.86

or 23 = a healthy BMI, or 154 ÷ 68.9² X 705 = 22.87 or 23 = a healthy BMI.

- A BMI of <19 indicates emaciation or underweight, 19-24 is healthy BMI, 25-29 is overweight and BMI 30-35 indicates obesity, and above 35 is an indication of extreme obesity.

How to calculate your Daily Energy Requirement (DER) Daily Energy Expenditure (DEE)?

Consumption of more than the daily energy requirement is the main cause of overweight, not a high fat diet, as everybody believes. The details have been explained in the chapters on CHO and lipids. Therefore, everybody will be interested to know their actual daily energy requirement. For this purpose, the American Dietetic Association has given **Mifflin-St Jeor** formulas for calculating the daily energy requirements. First, we have to calculate the Basal Energy Requirement (BER) as follows:

Men= 10 x weight in kg + 6.25 x height in cm - 5 x age in years + 5

Women= 10 x weight in kg + 6.25 x height in cm - 5 x age in years - 161

These calories are the basic calories needed for a bed ridden person, with zero physical activity i.e. BER. But every person will have some level of physical activity. So, to arrive at the actual calories needed, we have to multiply this BER with the **body activity factor**; which ranges from 1.2 to 1.9, depending on their physical activity.

1.2 to 1.4 = for persons with low physical activity or sedentary habits

1.5 to 1.6 = for persons with moderate physical activity

1.7 to 1.8 = for persons with high physical activity

1.9 = for sports persons

According to this formula, a 60-year-old man, weighing 70 kg, with 170 cm height and sedentary habits, the energy requirement will be:

(10X70 + 6.25X 170) – (5X60) +5 = 700+1062.5 or say 1063 =1763 - 300+5 = 1458 X 1.2 (sedentary) **= 1750 calories /day**

If the person is a woman, with the same data, then her daily calories requirements will be:

1763- 300-161= 1302 X 1.2= **1562 calories/day**.

This provides us the energy required/day. If we consume these calories daily, there will not be any weight gain or loss. If you want to lose body weight, 10-20% lesser calories may be consumed. Moreover, this calorie restriction must be gradual. Never go beyond 40% calorie restriction or a maximum of 500 calories cut per day. Restrict mainly CHO calories as far as possible, and never cut protein calories unless you have some kidney problem or under medical advice.

However, the major portion of excess dietary energy, whatever may be its source (CHO, lipids or proteins) will be converted into body fat, especially as saturated fat, since the human body cannot synthetize essential unsaturated fatty acids like PUFA. This will result in overweight and obesity. On the other hand, lower calorie consumption will utilize glycogen stored in the liver and muscles initially for energy, followed by depletion of body fat, and ultimately, body protein as body fuel (which happens only during starvation), resulting in weight loss, general weakness and low disease resistance capacity.

How to calculate your daily calorie consumption?
Once you know your DER, then your next question will be how to calculate and get the correct daily calorie consumption/requirement from the foods you eat. The question is simple, but the answer is complicated; because, unlike in domestic animals, we are consuming wide varieties of foods and the menu also varies daily. In the case of pets and livestock, we are giving one or two types of foods only and no daily change in menu. The calories are mentioned on the food packet, so it is very easy to dispense the right DER in the case of domestic animals.

In the case of humans, due to the wide variety of foods consumed, daily variations in the menu and quantities consumed and varied water levels in various foods, we cannot calculate the exact calories consumed daily. Some dietetics books, including ADA, USDA, NRC and this author's book on "Agro-forestry products," the nutrients' composition and calorific values of various foods and raw materials are given. In case of packaged foods, we can calculate the calories, based on the values on the label, but in case of fruits and vegetables, we cannot calculate the energy values so easily. If you know the quantities of CHO, lipids and proteins consumed daily on a dry matter basis (excluding water), you can calculate the daily energy consumed.

Daily Energy Consumed (DEC) = (grams of CHO + proteins consumed X 4) **+** (grams of lipids consumed X 9) **+** (grams /ml of alcohol in your drink X7).

Such calculation of DEC is not practicable for many people, so the most practicable way is, *do not over eat.* Check your body weight once a month. If there is an increase in body weight, your calorie consumption is higher. If there is 1 kg increase in body weight, it means roughly you have deposited 1 kg of extra fat in your body, which is equivalent to about 9,000 calories. If this weight gain happens in one month, then 9000 ÷ 30 days = 300 calories extra energy you have consumed/day, on an average. So in order to get rid of these extra calories, or body fat, you have three options.

1. Reduce 300 to 500 calories intake daily, mostly of refined CHO origin (about 100 to 150 g of lesser CHO /day), or

2. Burn these extra calories by doing extra physical work, or

3. Combine 1 and 2 methods above for quicker results, so that your body weight comes to normal level after one month.

Causes of obesity
There are many causes for obesity and overweight. Overeating alone may not be the only cause. Other causes are heredity, high calorie intake, especially of refined CHO origin, family history,

hormonal imbalance, especially hypothyroidism, eating calorie-rich junk foods, certain food additives present in junk foods, refined CHO, especially sugar rich foods like cookies, sweets, aerated-sweetened soft drinks, empty calorie foods, sedentary habits, lack of exercise and physical activity, use of anabolic steroid drugs, birth control pills and a combination of these factors.

Excess sugar and refined CHO are the most common causes of obesity

Among all the foods and food ingredients we eat, **sugar, refined CHO and foods having these two** are the most common causes of obesity and diabetes, if consumed in excess. Along with these two, many food additives and chemicals used in the food industry, especially in junk foods, will also cause several chronic diseases, including obesity. Even though the food additives are zero calorie chemicals and used in small quantities, many of them will interfere with the body's metabolism, resulting in body fat accumulation and overweight. Hence, they are unwanted foods for our body and health. They are the root cause for several chronic metabolic diseases like obesity, diabetes, elevated cholesterol, CVD, arthritis and many more. In fact, food manufacturers are secretly hiding this sugar in >80% of the foods we eat and drink, and it's one of key reasons for accumulation of fat in the abdomen and hip regions, resulting in obesity, diabetes and CVD. People are finding this abdominal fat nearly impossible to shed.

Many nutritionists have concluded that **sugar is eight times more addictive than cocaine and heroin.** It is inked to the deaths of almost 600,000 Americans a year. One recent study has found that almost all cookies, cakes, chocolates, ice creams, and sweets were as addictive forming as those of cocaine and heroin, because some addict-forming substances are incorporated in them. No wonder people have such a hard time saying "no" to sugary snack foods. They are designed to stimulate certain parts of your brain and create addictive behavior.

Sugar makes it nearly impossible to lose weight

Just a little bit of sugar can completely "short circuit" your efforts to lose weight. That's because sugar spikes your insulin levels. Insulin is the hormone that tells your body to store fat. In the presence of insulin, you cannot burn fat, says Dr. Eric Berg. "All of the fat-burning hormones are nullified when you have just a little bit of sugar." Even worse, excess sugar that isn't immediately converted into energy is converted into fat and stored in adipose tissue, which is very difficult to lose.

Sugar is present even in the so-called "healthy foods"

Many people who think they are being healthy with their food choices are shocked when they discover how much sugar they're actually consuming every day. This is because sugar is added to just about everything. For example, if a food label indicates it is 80% natural, the remaining 20% is mostly sugar and a few food additives. Pick up any loaf of bread at the grocery store and chances are you'll find sugar, honey, corn syrup, or brown rice syrup in the first five ingredients. But bread isn't the only food product that has added sugar. You'll find it in cookies, so called natural fruit juices, aerated drinks, crackers, cereals, yogurt, tomato sauce, even salad dressings and chips. Dr. Robert Lusting reported that out of >600,000 food items in the American grocery store, 80 percent have been spiked with added sugar, and the industry uses 56 other names for sugar on the label. Sugar is more addictive forming than heroin.

Cut out sugar and lose your body weight

The message is clear: Sugar causes the body to store fat and losing weight becomes a whole lot easier once you cut out sugar. In fact, these days the media is full of stories about popular celebrities cutting out sugar and losing weight. One of the most impressive success stories is Fergie, the Duchess of York, who lost 50 lbs. in just five months at the age of 54. Such an achievement would be impressive for a 30-year-old, but to lose 50 lbs. so quickly at 54 is, quite simply, amazing. If it worked for her, perhaps a similar no-sugar diet could help you achieve your weight loss goals, too. But how on earth do you get started when sugar is hidden in as much as 80% of the food you buy? It all starts with a quick lesson about which foods to eat and which to avoid. The best way to get rid of sugar is to prepare your own foods without sugar at home. Sugar is more harmful to obese persons than for diabetics.

Sugar substitutes and food additives

Do not use sugar substitutes, because they are more harmful than sugar, and many of them are carcinogenic. Stevia is a Japanese herb, having an active principle, 'stevioside.' It is said to be 100 to 300 times sweeter than sugar, but provides no calories and is safe. However, it is more commonly used in Japanese soft drinks, chewing gums and desserts to lower blood pressure by 10%, rather than as a sugar substitute.

Besides sugar and sugar substitutes, many food additives and chemicals present in aerated soft drinks and other junk foods also cause obesity or bring some metabolic changes in the body.

Bariatric nutrition - weight management - satiety- leptin & ghrelin

Leptin is a hormone produced by the adipose tissue (subcutaneous fat) that regulates energy balance by suppressing hunger/appetite. It is also called **satiety hormone** as well as **fat burning hormone.** It stimulates the hypothalamus in the brain to produce satiety, resulting in lesser consumption of food, leading to body weight control. **Egg protein, casein (milk protein) and isolated soy protein will stimulate leptin production, while high CHO diet suppresses leptin production.** On the other hand, **ghrelin,** another hormone, stimulates hunger, resulting in over-eating and obesity. Ghrelin is produced by the gastrointestinal track when it is empty or partially empty. Refined CHO rich foods also stimulate the secretion of ghrelin, because the GI track will be emptied quickly after a CHO rich diet.

Obesity is a multi-factorial and complex health issue, mainly controlled by leptin and ghrelin. Fasting and half-starving are not the answers for weight control. Fasting is good only during indigestion and stomach upset. During jaundice, high fever and complicated diseases, liquid diets are advisable. At the same time, feasting, especially consuming a high calorie diet must be avoided by all. If you have to feast occasionally, like at a marriage party, then skip the next one or two meals. Both fasting and feasting are not good for health.

Moreover, a program suitable for a few persons for weight reduction may not be suitable for others, due to individual variations. Current guidance for weight management encourages physical activity along with consuming an overall healthy eating pattern, which includes consumption of reduced energy whole grains, lean proteins, satiety foods like eggs, isolated soy and milk (casein) proteins, and negative calorie/zero calorie leafy vegetables and fruits.

A growing body of research suggests that dietary protein can help promote satiety, facilitating weight loss, when consumed as part of reduced energy diets. Several clinical trials have specifically assessed the effects of high-quality isolated protein from eggs, milk (casein) and soy protein on satiety and weight loss. For example:

- In a study in overweight adults, calorie-restricted diets that included either eggs or a bagel for breakfast were compared; the people who consumed eggs for breakfast lowered their body mass index by 61%, lost 65% more weight, and reported feeling more energetic than those who ate a bagel for breakfast.

- Men who consumed an egg breakfast versus a bagel breakfast showed that the **appetite hormone, ghrelin, was suppressed following eggs at breakfast, resulting in lesser food intake at lunch,** as was energy intake over the course of the day.

- A study of overweight pre-menopausal women that evaluated satiety responses to eating a turkey sausage, isolated milk/soya protein and/or egg breakfast sandwich versus a low-protein pancake breakfast showed better appetite control and fewer calories consumed at lunch following the egg-based breakfast.

- In another trial among subjects with type-2 diabetes, those who consumed two eggs per day, 15 g of isolated milk protein or soya protein for 6 days a week, reported lesser hunger and greater satiety than those who consumed CHO rich breakfast. It also resulted in weight loss and lesser HbA1c values.

- For weight reduction, consume 10 to 15 % lesser calories of CHO origin than recommended, or do extra exercise to burn the calories. But do not starve or skip any meal. Replace CHO and sugars with low calorie salads made up of mixed leafy vegetables, onions, cucumber etc. Do not use salad dressings having sugar; eat it raw or sprinkle on a little bit pepper. If you are not having BP, add little bit of salt also.

- Obese persons must consume a mixture of low calorie vegetables like cucumber, okra, various gourds, bell peppers, broccoli, asparagus, cluster beans, all leafy vegetables and low sugar fruits like guava, kiwi, berries etc. to an extent of 400 g/day, or about 25% of total calories.

- The restriction is only for calorie (energy) and not for other nutrients. Do not consume high glycemic index foods like sugar (or foods having added sugar), malt, refined flours, sweets, soft drinks and even sugar-added fruit juices. Energy restriction may not be effective for all obese persons.

- So more than the energy restriction, obese persons must consume food in such a way that 28-30% of the total calories comes from lipids, another 18-22% from protein sources (high protein diet), and only 40-50% comes from CHO source—that, too, from complex CHO, rich in fiber, like green leafy vegetable, fruits, whole grains and seeds (pulses), because fiber, lipids and protein rich foods take a long time for digestion and absorption, with low glycemic index. Persons having kidney function impairment and other metabolic problems must take high protein foods, based on the physician's advice only.

- For weight reduction, after lunch or dinner drink plain green tea, chamomile and many herbal teas, with lime juice but without sugar and milk.

- Consume daily at least 100 g of **negative calorie, zero calorie or fat burning foods**, also called **bariatric foods**, rich in fiber, like green leafy vegetables and low calorie fruits. For obese persons, the dietary fiber level may go up to a maximum of 60 g if there is no indigestion, stomach upset or any other problem.

- High calorie fruits like banana, apples, sapodilla (*sapota, chiku*), mango, dates and jackfruit are not suitable for weight reduction. Consume low calorie and less sweet fruits like guava, kiwi, various berries, oranges, grapefruit, grapes, wood apple and less common seasonal fruits.

- Chilled water also acts as a negative calorie food, because to bring this water to body temperature, some body calories will be consumed, but do not take too much chilled water, which may create some other health complications.

- Increase protein calories at the expense of CHO calories, proportionately.

- Reduce CHO-rich foods like grains, potato and tapioca in the food and increase low calorie vegetables and fruits. The reduction for obese persons are calories, CHO and total food consumption only, but not for micronutrients like vitamins and minerals, which supply "nil" energy. When an obese person cuts some portion of his food, he will be cutting that much portion of micronutrients also. Hence, to compensate this loss, he must take vitamin and mineral supplements to prevent any deficiency disease or breakdown of immunity

- In some obese persons, none of the above techniques will show considerable reduction in body weight/fat because the body fat reserve will remain undisturbed, even during starvation and low calorie diets, where the body glycogen and muscle protein will be utilized for energy purpose. The later source is not desirable because it will make the person weak. So, **to initiate/mobilize body fat to burn for energy purpose, take CHO-free-low calorie food for 1-2 weeks, or until 3-5 kg reduction in body weight, due to burning of body fat for energy purpose. After this body fat mobilization has started, low calorie food may be consumed to supply calories from CHO: fats + oils: proteins at 50:30:20 ratios**. The first CHO-free-low calorie diet must be derived from very low glycemic index foods like sugar-free yogurts, eggs, meats, soy protein, whey, all leafy vegetables and low-calorie-high-fiber vegetables and fruits like berries. Such diet shall not include any grains, tubers (potato etc.), nuts, seeds, bakery products, sugar + starch rich fruits (like banana, dates, jackfruit, apple etc.).

Herbs and spices that reduce body weight

There are many spices and herbs which can reduce the body weight, if efficiently utilized. Some of them are available in the market in capsule and powder forms.

1. *Garcinia cambogia* is a native plant of Southeast Asia, also grown in India. Its fruits look like small sized pumpkins. It is capable of suppressing appetite, burning calories and reducing body weight by maintaining negative calorie balance.

2. *Psidium guajava:* **Guava** is a widely cultivated fruit in all tropical countries. Its fruits and leaves have the active principles, nerdidiol, sitosterol, leucocyanidin, caryophyllene, β-bisaboline and p-selinene. They are powerful antioxidants, anti-inflammatory and anti-bacterial agents. Regular consumption of these fruits and leaves helps in body weight loss, diabetes control and reduces cholesterol, hypertension, sugar and diarrhea.

3. Vegetables and spices belonging to the ***crucifaciae*** family, such as broccoli, Brussels sprouts, cabbage, cauliflower,

choy, kale, lettuce, mustard, turnip etc. contain active principles-phytonutrients, indole-3-carbinol, which help to reduce the abdominal fat by burning calories and reducing body weight.

4. Mushrooms, especially red mushrooms of Japan and China, are low calorie food and contain the active principle, muscarin, which will burn the calories and keep you slim. Moreover, they will reduce BP, blood sugar, cancer, cholesterol and TGL.

5. All **leafy vegetables** are **fiber rich** and **negative calorie foods**. For their digestion and utilization, some calories have to be utilized, as explained in the chapter on dietary fiber. Daily consumption of 50-100 g of fresh leafy vegetables will not only keep you trim, but also prevent constipation and keep diabetes, TGL and cholesterol under check.

6. There are several other weight reducing herbs and spices. All negative calorie foods and fiber rich foods listed in the chapters on CHO and fiber, and many herbs listed in the chapter on herbs and spices, are useful for body weight reduction.

7. Herbs like nettle leaves, guarana, cayenne pepper (red pepper, black/white pepper, all bell peppers), dandelions, *Coleus forskohlii*, gymnema silvesta, hoodia gordonii, fennel, yerba mate, sea weed-kelp, mustard, ginseng, turmeric, psyllium, acai berry have lipid lowering properties.

8. Drink **green tea** alone or in combination with hibiscus, mint, ginger, cinnamon, cardamom, chameleon, dandelion, marigold petals, **without** any sugar, sugar-substitutes or milk, for weight reduction.

9. Reduce the calories of CHO and lipids origin, but do not cut protein calories. For weight reduction purpose, the food calories of CHO—lipids, protein origin—must preferably be in the 50: 30: 20 ratios, but the total calories must not exceed the recommended levels. This ratio will also work well for diabetic patients.

Check with your physician to find out the exact cause of obesity, especially non-dietary causes like hormonal imbalance, hypo-thyroidism, menstrual problem, low BMR/RMR, heredity, insufficient physical activity or over appetite, and follow the guidelines given by the physician. Find out the exact cause(s) for obesity, and then take suitable steps to reduce the body weight. In case of none of the above dietary techniques and physical exercise are working to reduce the body weight, for those whose BMI is >30, and in persons whose appetite is high, **bariatric surgery** may be performed, based on the recommendation of the surgeon. Two types of surgeries are performed; namely:

- 1. **Gastric band surgery**: reduces the stomach size, result-ing in lesser food intake.

- 2. **Gastric sleep surgery:** Here the **ghrelin** secreting tissues are removed. **Ghrelin** is an appetite-increasing hormone. If this is removed, appetite will be suppressed, resulting in reduced food intake and weight reduction.

In conclusion, to overcome overweight and obesity, consume varieties of fresh, unprocessed fiber rich, low calorie whole foods, especially low in CHO calories. Eat fresh low calorie/ negative calorie vegetables/fruits and satiety foods like eggs. Do sufficient exercise and walking to burn fat. Take the suggestions of a bariatric specialist to find out exact reasons and remedies for overweight.

Chapter 17

Dietary Methods to Control Diabetes

Diabetes mellitus is the fastest growing metabolic/endocrine disorder in the world. More than 20% of the persons in the world over 30 years of age are diabetic. There are type-1 and type-2 diabetes and also other types. Type-1 starts from childhood. Even type-2 starts as early as 15 years of age. As such, it is the number one disease in the world. India has the fastest growing incidences of diabetes in the world. About 18.5% of the world's diabetics are in India. The actual figure must be still higher than this, because millions of poor people, in developing countries, especially in the rural areas suffer from diabetes silently, without undergoing any treatment, due to poverty and ignorance. Hence, they are not included in this list of diabetics. Every year millions of new diabetics are added, but none of them are getting rid of the disease because no treatment is available at present to cure diabetes. All the drugs available are only to control the blood sugar level and other secondary complications. Once a person suffers from diabetes, he/she will continue to be diabetic until the rest of his/her life.

What causes diabetes?
Diabetes is an endocrine disorder, where the pancreas is unable to produce enough insulin needed to regulate blood and tissue sugar levels. Insulin is needed for the cells to take up enough sugar for their function. In the absence—or insulin insufficiency—cells cannot take enough sugar, resulting in shooting up of blood sugar. Sometimes the cells are resistant to insulin and sugar builds up in

the blood. Since the cells do not have enough sugar, they cannot function properly and they become weak. This **excess blood sugar** will cause inflammation of the arteries, and **trans-fatty acids and free radicals**, as reported in earlier chapters, will act as abrasive materials and damage the arterial walls, LDLC will deposit over the damaged arterial walls and block the free flow of blood, causing CVD. Thus, the diabetes will predispose the diabetics to CVD.

Heredity or family history is one of the prime causes for diabetes. Persons whose close relatives are diabetic will have more chances to become diabetic, but it doesn't mean that they will definitely get it. If they are precautious, by following an active lifestyle, eating whole foods with enough fiber, and avoiding sugar rich junk foods, they can easily escape from diabetes. Obese persons are more prone for diabetes than persons with normal BMI.

Due to several global changes reported in Chapter Two, like pollution, junk fast foods rich in calories, especially from sugars and refined and polished CHO, insufficient fiber in the diet, lack of physical work, sedentary life style, obesity, irregular food habits, overeating, chronic alcoholism, smoking, excess abdominal fat, and emotional stress are other predisposing causes for diabetes.

Glycemic index

The glycemic index (GI) is a measure of the blood glucose-raising potential of the carbohydrate content of a food compared to a reference food, namely pure glucose. Carbohydrate-containing foods can be classified as high (≥70), moderate (56-69), or low-GI (≤55) foods, relative to pure glucose (GI=100). The concept of glycemic index (GI) has thus been developed in order to rank dietary carbohydrates based on their overall effect on postprandial blood glucose concentration relative to pure glucose. The GI represents the relative quality of a carbohydrate-containing food. The GI of selected carbohydrate-containing foods can be found in **Table 17-1.**

Consumption of high-GI foods causes a sharp increase in postprandial blood glucose concentration that declines rapidly, whereas consumption of low-GI foods results in a lower blood glucose concentration that declines gradually. The glycemic load (GL) is obtained by multiplying the quality of carbohydrates in a given food (GI) by the amount of carbohydrates in a serving of that food. Prospective cohort studies found high GI or GL diets to be associated with a higher risk of adverse health outcomes, including type-2 diabetes mellitus and cardiovascular disease.

In the past, doctors and dieticians advised their patients to eat less simple (sugars) and more complex carbohydrates (polysaccharides), assuming that consuming starchy foods would lead to smaller increases in blood glucose than simple sugars. This assumption turned out to be too simplistic, since the blood glucose (glycemic) response to complex carbohydrates has been found to vary considerably.

Meta-analyses of observational studies have found little-to-no evidence of an association between high dietary GI and GL and risk of cancer. Lowering the GL of the diet may be an effective method to improve glycemic control in individuals with type-2 diabetes mellitus. This approach is not currently included in the overall strategy of diabetes management. Several dietary intervention studies found that low-GI/GL diets were as effective as conventional, low-fat diets in reducing body weight. Both types of diets resulted in beneficial effects on metabolic markers associated with the risk of type-2 diabetes mellitus and cardiovascular disease.

Table-17-1 Glycemic index (GI) and Glycemic loads (GL) of certain foods

Food	GI (Glucose = 100)	CHO in 100 g	GL =GI X CHO ÷ 100 (= GI of glucose)
Sugar	83	98	81.3
Potato, boiled	82	60	49.2
Sweets, ice cream, chocolates	82	40	32.8
Corn flakes, popcorn	79	60	47.4
Cookies, cakes, crackers, wafers	78	64	49.9

Doughnut, muffin,	76	68	51.7
Watermelon	76	12	9.1
Soft drinks	74	15	11.1
White bread & bun	74	32	23.7
White rice, boiled	68	24	16.3
Brown rice, boiled	63	24	15.1
French fries, chips	63	78	49.1
Dates, jackfruit	62	36	22.3
Parota, Nan (flat bread using refined flour)	62	62	38.4
Honey	58	78	45.2
Mango, sapodilla	58	20	11.6
Banana, large	55	24	13.2
Pineapple, papaya, grapes	54	14	7.6
Wheat chappathi (flat bread)	52	62	32.2
Spaghetti/pasta-white, boiled	46	28	12.9
Whole-grain bread	46	30	13.8
All-bran cereal	45	22	9.9
Spaghetti/pasta whole-meal, boiled	32	27	8.7
Orange, nectarine	42	11	4.6
Apple, apricot, berries	39	16	6.2
Pear, kiwi, guava	38	14	5.3
Milk	33	4	1.3
Carrots, beet, radish, turnip	33	14	4.6
Okra, cluster beans, green beans, gourds	29	12	3.5
Beans, lentils boiled	28	18	5.0
Barley, oats, millets, quinoa boiled	28	19	5.3
Cashews, almonds, walnuts	25	30	7.5
Peanuts, peas, chick peas, pulses	18	25	4.5
Eggs	9	1	0.09
Fish & meats	7	0	0.0

Data in Table-17-1 indicates that whole grains have lesser GI than polished grains (white flours). Nuts, eggs, meats, oats, quinoa and millets have low GI and GL values. Hence, these foods are preferred for diabetics. White, polished, refined grains; sweets, cookies, crackers, chocolates, cakes, soft drinks, bottled fruit juices with added sugar and other junk foods made up of refined CHO, including sugar have the highest GI and GL, such foods are not only harmful for diabetics, but also for others. Hence, consumption of such junk foods must be avoided or restricted.

Whether low-GI foods could improve overall blood glucose control in people with type 1 or type 2 diabetes mellitus has been investigated in a number of intervention studies. A meta-analysis of 19 randomized controlled trials that included 840 diabetic patients (191 with type 1 diabetes and 649 with type 2 diabetes) found that consumption of low-GI foods improved short-term and long-term control of blood glucose concentrations, reflected by significant decreases in fructosamine and glycosylated hemoglobin (HbA1c) levels. However, these results need to be cautiously interpreted because of significant heterogeneity among the included studies. The American Diabetes Association has rated poorly the current evidence supporting the substitution of low-GL foods for high-GL foods to improve glycemic control in adults with type 1 or type 2 diabetes. Well-controlled studies are needed to further assess whether the use of low-GI/GL diets could significantly improve long-term glycemic control and the quality of life of subjects with diabetes. However, it is better to consume low GI foods, both by diabetics and pre-diabetics to control diabetes, as well as by non-diabetics to prevent the occurrence of diabetes.

The glycosylated hemoglobin A1c test (**HbA1c**) is a laboratory test which reveals average blood glucose levels over a period of two to three months. Specifically, it measures the number of glucose molecules attached to hemoglobin in red blood cells. The test takes advantage of the lifecycle of red blood cells. Although constantly replaced, individual cells live for about four months, so by measuring attached glucose in a current blood sample, average blood sugar levels over the previous two to three months can be determined. The HbA1c values equivalent to the conventional blood sugar values in mg/dl are reported in **Table-17.2** for reference. The HbA1c test results are expressed as a percentage, with 4 to 6 % considered as normal. Persons with values of 6 to 6.9 are considered as pre-diabetic and those 7 and above HbA1c values are considered as diabetic.

Table-17-2: Glycosylated Hemoglobin A1c test (HbA1c) equivalent to blood glucose levels (mg/100ml)

HbA1c	4.0	4.1	4.2	4.3	4.4	4.5	4.6	4.7	4.8	4.9
Glucose	68	71	74	77	80	82	85	88	91	94
HbA1c	5.0	5.1	5.2	5.3	5.4	5.5	5.6	5.7	5.8	5.9
Glucose	97	100	103	105	108	111	114	117	120	123
HbA1c	6.0	6.1	6.2	6.3	6.4	6.5	6.6	6.7	6.8	6.9
Glucose	125	128	131	134	137	140	143	146	148	151
HbA1c	7.0	7.1	7.2	7.3	7.4	7.5	7.6	7.7	7.8	7.9
Glucose	154	157	160	163	166	169	171	174	177	180
HbA1c	8.0	8.1	8.2	8.3	8.4	8.5	8.6	8.7	8.8	8.9
Glucose	183	186	189	192	194	197	200	203	206	209
HbA1c	9.0	9.1	9.2	9.3	9.4	9.5	9.6	9.7	9.8	9.9
Glucose	212	214	217	220	223	226	229	232	235	237
HbA1c	10.0	10.1	10.2	10.3	10.4	10.5	10.6	10.7	10.8	10.9
Glucose	240	243	246	249	252	255	258	260	263	266
HbA1c	11.0	11.1	11.2	11.3	11.4	11.5	11.6	11.7	11.8	11.9
Glucose	269	272	275	278	280	283	286	289	292	295
HbA1c	12.0	12.1	12.2	12.3	12.4	12.5	12.6	12.7	12.8	12.9
Glucose	298	301	303	306	309	312	315	318	321	324
HbA1c	13.0	13.1	13.2	13.3	13.4	13.5	13.6	13.7	13.8	13.9
Glucose	326	329	332	335	338	341	344	346	349	352

Dietary methods to control diabetes

- Lowering dietary GL can be achieved by increasing the consumption of foods having low GI, like whole grains, especially millets, quinoa, oats and barley, eggs, fish, lean meats, nuts, legumes, leafy vegetables and by decreasing intakes of moderate and high GI foods like potatoes, all foods having added sugar, white rice, white bread, and soft drinks.

- The problems of elevated blood glucose level, hyper-cholesterolemia, TGL, diabetes and pre-diabetes can be reduced if junk foods consumption is stopped. As stated earlier, a healthy man with sedentary habits needs about 2000 K. calories of energy/day, and a healthy woman with sedentary habits needs about 1,700 K. calories/day, which is roughly equivalent to about 30 cal./kg body weight/day. However, overweight and obese persons shall consume <25 cal./kg/day. On the other hand, growing children, sports persons, pregnant and lactating women need >30 cal./kg /day. The details of calculation of exact energy requirements are discussed in the chapter on obesity management.

- As per the dietary guidelines—RDA recommended by various countries—in a healthy adult's diet, these **daily recommended calories must be obtained from CHO, lipids and proteins, in the ideal ratio of 60:27:13** respectively, as reported in earlier chapters. However, **for diabetics, the ideal recommended calorie ratio will be in the range of 50-54: 30-33: 14-18, from CHO, lipids and proteins, depending on other complications they have**. Unfortunately, this actual ratio in India is 73, 17:10, as shown in Table-5-1, 2 & 3. This ratio is more diabeto-genic, as well as deficient in essential amino acids and fatty acids. Moreover, in India the middle and high income group consume more than the required calories, especially from refined starch, polished rice, hydrogenated fat (vanaspathi-Dalda) and sugars like all bakery products, sweets, paratta, pastas, noodles, burgers and other restaurant fast foods. Hence, all such diabeto-genic foods must be avoided.

- Additionally, the consumption of high-GI foods that are low in cereal fiber was associated with a 59% increase in diabetes risk, compared to low-GI and high-cereal-fiber foods. High-GL and low-cereal-fiber diets were associated with a 47% increase in risk compared to low-GL and high-cereal-fiber diets. Hence, it is advisable for diabetic and non-diabetic to consume fiber rich, low calorie foods.

- Non-vegetarian diabetics must consume 1 or 2 eggs, 50-100 g fish (with skin) + 50 g skinless chicken + 250 - 400 ml milk (without added sugar) per day, along with legumes, pulses, lentils, multiple whole grain foods, green leafy vegetables (without any ready-made salad dressings—some olive oil + spices can be used, but not sugar and salt) and low sugar fruits, depending on their budget.

- Eggs + fish + meats/nuts + leafy vegetables + legumes + whole grain food combinations are the best for diabetes patients. However, strict watch must be placed so not to exceed the total calories needed for them.

- Lacto-ovo vegetarians can consume 1 or 2 eggs + 400-500 ml milk (without added sugar) per day, along with extra legumes, nuts, pulses, lentils, multiple whole grain foods, green leafy vegetables (without any ready-made salad dressings—some olive oil + spices can be used, but not sugar and salt) and low sugar fruits, depending on their budget. If eggs are not used (lacto-vegetarian) 25 g of tofu/cheese + additional 60 g of nuts and pulses may be consumed.

- Vegans (no animal products) can take up extra pulses, legumes, sesame, mixed nuts, especially walnuts, flax seeds, hemp seeds, chia seeds etc. to supply O-3 FA, soya chunks/protein, plus usual vegetables, greens and whole grains. Since vegetarian foods are deficient in vitamin-D,

B12, essential amino acids (EAA) like methionine, lysine and few minerals, they have to take daily multi-vitamin and mineral supplements as per RDA. No need to take it at therapeutic dose. Sesame seeds will supply the EAA methionine, and soya will supply the EAA lysine. They must also take probiotic capsule on alternate days.

- Obese diabetic persons must consume the same foods as above, but they must cut their daily calories to about 80 % of their requirement and increase the fiber levels to an additional 10 g, i.e. about 50 – 55 g/day. If they feel that the fiber diet is causing indigestion and stomach upset, they can reduce it to 40-45 g/day.

- While consuming high fiber diets, some micronutrients like vitamins and minerals may be adsorbed with fiber and eliminated. Hence, multivitamin and mineral supplements are essential.

- Do not use sugar substitutes, because they are more harmful than sugar and many of them are carcinogenic. Besides sugar and sugar substitutes, many food additives and chemicals present in aerated soft drinks and other junk foods also cause obesity, which may cause over consumption or bring some metabolic changes in the body.

- Conclusions from several recent meta-analyses of prospective studies suggest that low-GI and GL diets might have a modest but significant effect in the prevention of type-2 diabetes. Organizations like Diabetes UK and the European Association for the Study of Diabetes have included the use of diets of low GI/GL and high in dietary fiber and whole grains in their recommendations for diabetes prevention in high-risk individuals.

- A randomized controlled weight loss trial in people with diagnosed type 2 diabetes showed improved lipid and glucose markers following consumption of 2 eggs per day for 12 weeks. An egg-based breakfast produces satiety and promotes glycemic control in people with type-2 diabetes and pre-diabetes, as compared to a high-carbohydrate breakfast. Egg is also rich in protein with negligible CHO. Hence, egg is an ideal food for diabetics and pre-diabetes, as well as for obese persons, because it has high biological value protein, essential emulsified lipids and causes satiety, which suppresses appetite and prevents overeating.

Herbs and spices to control diabetes:

- Certain herbs are very specific for diabetes and used in Ayurveda system of medicine to cure diabetes. Gurmar/chakkara kolli (sugar killer) or gymnema sylvestreor, Tinospora cordifolia etc. These herbs will stimulate the pancreas to secrete more insulin. Herbs and spices suitable for obese persons are also suitable for diabetic patients. For details of the herbs and spices to be consumed, refer to Chapter Thirteen, Herbs and Spices, as well as Chapter Sixteen, Obesity and Weight Management. Certain vegetables (like bitter gourd) and spices (like fenugreek) have active principles like chromium, methyl hydroxyl chalcone polymer (MHCP), which will stimulate the pancreas to secrete more insulin.

- Neem (Azardiracta indica) leaf or flower powder = 2-3 g/day or neem oil = 1 ml /day, will keep the blood sugar under control.

- Organic chromium, methyl hydroxyl chalcone polymer (MHCP), corsolic acid and gymnemic acid, present in gymnema sylvestreor, fenugreek seeds, bitter gourd, neem, banana leaf extract, will control blood sugar levels and diabetes.

- In diabetic patients, the islets of Langerhans in the pancreas are not secreting enough insulin needed to control blood sugar, which is due to formation of a fatty layer around the pancreas and fatty infiltration. If this fatty layer and fatty infiltration is removed surgically or by using some medicines, before the tissues are fully damaged, they will start secreting the insulin, and the persons will be free from diabetes. Herbs like Eclypta alba, phyllanthus neruri, Terminalia chebula, gymnema sylvestreor, Tinospora cordifolia, Indian gooseberry, fenugreek etc., if taken at early stage of diabetes for two months, can reverse the insulin secretion.

- Avoid all junk foods, especially those having sugars, sugar substitutes (these sugar substitutes are more dangerous than sugar), processed foods, soft drinks, cakes, sweets and other high calorie foods. Take whole, least processed or unprocessed foods, like fresh fruits and vegetables, especially leafy vegetables.

- In a diabetes patient's diet, about 10% must be leafy vegetables + 15-20% other mixed vegetables + 15-25% fresh low-sugar, low calorie mixed fruits + 10% mixed nuts, lentils, beans, peas and pulses + <20-25% whole cereals + the remaining will be milk, eggs, fish, chicken or extra vegetable protein sources.

- Along with the proper diet, dietary habits are equally important. Take food 5 to 6 times a day (split feeding), instead of 3 or lesser number of times, but each meal must be in small quantities. Of these, one mealtime food will be only fruits, because fruits cannot be combined with regular meals. The total calories in all the foods consumed in a day must not exceed the recommended calories for the person, as suggested in the previous chapters on carbohydrates and obesity.

Non-dietary methods

Physical work and exercise are major steps to control blood sugar levels and diabetes. Have a brisk walk for 30 - 60 minutes daily + yoga, meditation, breathing exercise, gym or stretching exercises for 30 minutes, depending on your age and other health problems. By proper diet management, as mentioned above, combined with walking, yoga and exercise, diabetes can be kept under control with the least number of drugs, or even no drugs. However, blood glucose levels and other tests must be checked, as per doctors' advice.

Herbal supplements, healthy food habits, walking, yoga, meditation, breathing exercise, swimming, suitable exercise, active-positive-disciplined lifestyle, minimizing mental stress, avoiding smoking and adequate sleep will supplement and compliment the medication, if any, as per the doctor's advice, and will prevent, cure or keep under control all chronic metabolic diseases and conditions like diabetes, obesity, CVD, LDLC, TGL and hypertension.

Chapter 18

Dietary Methods to Control CVD and Cholesterol

Cardiovascular diseases (CVD) include all ailments to the heart and blood vessels—that's the circulatory system. It includes blood pressure (BP high or low) high cholesterol, high triglycerides (TGL), ischemic heart disease, heart attack, stroke, internal bleeding, cardiac fibrillation, arterial blocks, cardiac insufficiency and many more ailments. About 30% of all deaths in India and 1 in 3 deaths in USA are due to CVD. As per WHO, it is the number one killer disease in the world. High blood pressure is a chronic disease that affects more than 75 million people in the United States, according to the AHA report. More than 40% of the world's population over 40 years of age suffers from high BP and other CVD. Very few are suffering from low BP. Both are not good, but high BP is more dangerous. As per another survey in Europe, more than one-third of adults are suffering from CVD, obesity, overweight, diabetes and other metabolic diseases. Moreover, this figure is going up year after year.

Indians are having higher incidences of diabetes, >LDLC, <HDLC, cardiovascular diseases, in spite of very low lipids and cholesterol consumption, because of excess consumption of calories from refined starchy foods, sugar and sweets, which will be deposited as saturated body fat, especially as abdominal fat. If the calorie intake is within the recommended levels (2000 cal. for men & 1700 cal. for

women of average body weight and sedentary habits), the entire calories will be burnt and fat deposition will not take place. So the culprit is excess calories and not excess fat or cholesterol. For more details, refer to several earlier chapters.

Why CVD and other chronic diseases are more prevalent now?
The main reasons for this ever-growing catastrophe are mentioned in the earlier chapters. Environment, air, water and food pollution, adulteration, sugar, salt, refined fast foods, junk foods having thousands of harmful chemicals, change in lifestyle, sedentary habits, lack of physical work, faulty food habits, imbalanced foods, lack of dietary fiber, too many food additives—many of which are harmful to the health—emotional stress, drug misuse, chronic alcoholism, and smoking are common causes for all these diseases, as mentioned earlier. All these causes will not produce CVD and other diseases overnight or in a short period; it may take a few decades. Moreover, these predisposing causes are synergistic, cumulative and additive in nature, so one must be careful to avoid these chronic diseases by avoiding the above predisposing causes.

Cardio-metabolic health
Cardio-metabolic health is a relatively new term that encompasses cardiovascular and metabolic diseases, including type-2 diabetes, obesity, and metabolic syndrome. **In fact, CVD, obesity and diabetes are interrelated. Obese persons are more likely to get CVD and diabetes and the vice versa is also true**. Collectively, such conditions are the leading cause of preventable deaths worldwide. They all share similar risk factors like overweight/obesity, high LDLC, TGL, and hypertension, which can be modified by diet and lifestyle choices.

Still, many people believe that dietary cholesterol will increase serum cholesterol. Even some doctors and dieticians in developing countries like India are advising their patients to avoid cholesterol foods like eggs. In the earlier chapter on cholesterol, it has been clearly demonstrated, with many scientific evidences, that there is no correlation between dietary and serum cholesterols. The available evidence indicates that eggs, when consumed as part of an overall healthy diet pattern, do not affect risk factors for cardio-metabolic disease.

Recent recommendations from the American Heart Association, American College of Cardiology and American Diabetes Association, CNS, EFSA, ION, MRFIT etc. do not limit egg or cholesterol intake, a recent change from earlier guidance from these organizations. In fact, several global health organizations, including Health Canada, the Canadian Heart and Stroke Foundation, the Australian Heart Foundation and the Irish Heart Foundation, promote eggs as part of a heart-healthy diet. Given the public health significance of understanding cardio-metabolic diseases, research on risk reduction remains an active area of pursuit.

A randomized controlled study in people with metabolic syndrome showed that those consuming two whole eggs per day for breakfast, as part of a reduced carbohydrate diet, experienced favorable changes in HDL-cholesterol, insulin sensitivity, and other aspects of the lipoprotein lipid profile.

Glycemic index and CVD
Numerous observational studies have examined the relationship between dietary GI/GL (glycemic index & glycemic load) and the incidence of cardiovascular events, especially coronary heart disease (CHD) and stroke. A meta-analysis of 14 prospective cohort studies (229,213 participants, mean follow-up of 11.5 years) found a 13% and 23% increased risk of cardiovascular disease (CVD) with high versus low dietary GI and GL, respectively. Three independent meta-analyses of prospective studies also reported that higher GI or GL was associated with increased risk of CHD. A recent analysis of the European Prospective Investigation into cancer and nutrition (EPIC) study in 20,275 Greek participants, followed for a median of 10.4 years, showed a significant increase in CHD incidence and mortality with high dietary GL, specifically in those with high BMI (≥28). This is in line with earlier findings in the Nurses' Health Study (NHS) showing that a high dietary GL was associated with a doubling of the risk of CHD over 10 years in women with higher (35)

vs. lower BMI (23). A similar finding was reported in a cohort of middle-aged Dutch women followed for nine years.

Additionally, high dietary GL (but not GI) was associated with a 19% increased risk of stroke in pooled analyses of prospective cohort studies. A meta-analysis of seven prospective studies (242,132 participants; 3,255 stroke cases) found that dietary GL was associated with an overall 23% increase in risk of stroke and a specific 35% increase in risk of ischemic stroke; GL was not found to be related to hemorrhagic stroke. Overall, observational studies have found that higher glycemic load diets are associated with increased risk of cardiovascular disease, especially in women and in those with higher BMI.

Dietary methods to control CVD, cholesterol and TGL

- All dietary methods to reduce obesity, overweight, cholesterol, TGL, CVD and diabetes are interrelated. Reduction of total calorie intake, especially calories of refined CHO origin, sugar, salt, junk foods and refined fast foods, increasing the dietary fiber to 30-40 g/day, as detailed in the chapter on fiber, and doing exercise, walking, and change in lifestyle are a few steps to get rid of CVD, TGL, LDLC, diabetes and obesity.

- As mentioned in earlier chapters, especially in Chapter Thirteen on herbs and spices, several condiments, spices and herbs are very effective to reduce blood pressure, cholesterol and triglycerides, without any side effects. Herbs can help your circulation and heart by widening and relaxing blood vessels to prevent damage. Herbs can also help prevent clots and blockages forming in the blood vessels. **Herbs that lower the blood pressure are** *Eclipta Alba* (Bringaraj), Indian gooseberry (amla), aswagandha, ginseng, *Cassia augustifolia* (Swarna pathri), *phylanthus neruri*, arogya pacha, dandelion, spirulina, azola, alfalfa, clover, soy protein and many more.

- Consume **heart and blood vessels friendly condiments and spices** like, cinnamon, ginger, garlic, basil, holy basil, white basil, onion, cardamom, cloves, turmeric, bay leaves, black pepper, white pepper, red pepper, coriander, fenugreek, cumin, mustard, aniseeds, saffron, oregano, rosemary, dill and many more, having heart friendly active principles, as shown in Chapter Thirteen Tables. They will reduce blood pressure and keep the arteries healthy. They also reduce LDL cholesterol and TGL. Therefore, have spicy foods, having many spices, but avoid sugar and reduce salt (sodium). Enjoy spicy and heart-friendly foods. Since we are using condiments and spices in small quantities and they are rich in fiber, the energy contribution by them is insignificant and ignorable.

- Consume vegetables good for the heart, like all leafy vegetables, celery, beets, green pepper, bell pepper, all gourds, cucumber, cabbage, cauliflower, broccoli, okra, lettuce, kale and many more, which are very rich in potassium, calcium, magnesium, which will reduce BP, LDLC and TGL.

- Consume fresh fruits like grapes, especially red grapes, guava, watermelon, tender coconut water, kiwi, all berries, apple, banana, oranges, mango, papaya, sapodilla, peaches, nectarines, wood apple, apricot, cranberries, and many more, which are rich in potassium, magnesium, which will reduce BP, LDLC and TGL.

- Wash all vegetables, fruits and leaves thoroughly under running water, before cutting, to remove dirt, waxes, pesticides, herbicides and other chemicals.

- Use fresh fruits and vegetables as much as possible instead of canned, frozen and preserved foods and juices, which may have some preservatives and have lost their active principles to some extent.

- Consume seeds and nuts rich in omega-3 fatty acids, potassium and magnesium, like flax seeds (linseed), chia seeds, walnuts, almonds, cashews, pistachios and pine and hemp seeds. Since they have high oil levels, with high calories, consume them to about 10-20 g/day only. Consume two or more varieties, instead of one. Vegetarians, especially vegans can consume nuts up to 30 g/day, depending on the other foods and their health status.

- Peas, chickpea, mung bean, green lentil, red lentil, pinto bean, kidney bean, and other beans and lentils are low in oils but rich in proteins and fiber. Hence, these foods must be included, about 30 g daily and higher levels for vegetarians and vegans.

- Oil and protein rich foods like sesame, peanuts, soya must be consumed to a limited extent, replacing CHO, because they have low glycemic index and are suitable for diabetes patients.

- Use cooking oils recommended in the chapter on lipids. Preferably use a blended oil having 15-20% SFA + 40-45% MUFA (O-9) + 30-40% O-6 PUFA +3-5% O-3 PUFA, for healthy heart and blood vessels. On example of best-blended oil will be, olive oil = 30% + coconut or palm oil = 18% + canola oil = 30% + rice bran oil = 20% + flax seed/hemp seed/walnut oil = 2%, which will supply the above ideal fatty acids ratio. Alternatively, use different oils during breakfast, lunch and dinner preparations.

- Minerals good for heart and blood vessels are potassium and magnesium (both present in many fruits and vegetables). **Consider boosting potassium.** Potassium can lessen the effects of sodium on blood pressure. The best source of potassium is fruits and vegetables, rather than supplements. Talk to your doctor about the potassium level that is best for you, which is usually about 4000 mg/day.

- Nutritionally, alcohol can be both good and bad for your health. In small amounts, it can potentially lower your blood pressure by 2 to 4 mm Hg. But that protective effect is lost if you drink too much alcohol. Generally, no more than one drink a day for women and for men older than age 65, and no more than two a day for men age 65 and younger. One drink equals to 12 ounces of beer, five ounces of wine or 1.5 ounces of 80-proof liquor. These drinks are equivalent to total 100% absolute ethyl alcohol level of 12 and 24 ml/day for women and men, respectively. Of these alcoholic drinks, red wine is better, because it is rich in lycopene and resveratrol, which are powerful antioxidants, and they reduce serum TGL and increase good HDLC, to some extent. Drinking more than moderate amounts of alcohol can actually raise blood pressure by several points. It can also reduce the effectiveness of blood pressure medications. Moreover, alcohol is habit forming. **Hence, it is better to avoid alcoholic drinks**.

- Stevia is an herb, having an active principle, stevioside. It is said to be 100 to 300 times sweeter than sugar, but provides no calories. Stevia has also been hailed as a blood pressure buster. Stevia is commonly used in Japanese soft drinks, chewing gums and desserts. It can lower blood pressure by 10% when given at a dose of 250 mg, three times daily.

- Herbs like barberry, goldenseal and Oregon grape, contain a chemical called berberine. It is effective to treat both high cholesterol and high blood pressure, making it a real benefit to a healthy heart.

- Drinking just a cup of fresh **beetroot juice** daily can have amazing effects on your heart health. Scientists have found that the nitrate and potassium content in beetroot juice provides benefits for blood pressure.

- **Cayenne pepper** (common green/red chili) is probably the fastest acting food to lower blood pressure. It can be taken along with other spices in the ratio mentioned following in this chapter.

- **Coconut Water:** This natural beverage assists in the overall maintenance of good cardiovascular health. Research has shown that those suffering from high blood pressure generally have low potassium levels. Coconut water is rich in potassium, which allows it to help manage blood pressure in the body.

- **Almonds, walnuts & pine nuts:** These nuts have a few heart healthy components, such as flavonoids, potassium, and omega-3 fatty acids. Flavonoids and omega-3's have been proven to promote cardiovascular health, and potassium (as mentioned above) helps regulate blood pressure. The MUFA found in almonds lower blood cholesterol levels as well as reduce arterial inflammation, which ultimately lowers blood pressure.

- **Turmeric:** the active principle in turmeric is known as curcumin, which will drastically decrease inflammation throughout the body and protects the arteries and other tissues. It also reduces hypertension.

- **Fresh lime juice** is rich in Vitamin-C and other anti-oxidants, as well as other health promoting components. It is very effective in reducing cholesterol, sugar, obesity and BP, if consumed at 2-3 ml/day, but salt and sugar must not be added. About 5 ml of pure honey may be added, but it is not compulsory. For better results, take it with other synergistic ingredients, as mentioned below.

- **Ginger + turmeric + cinnamon + cardamom + chili (red pepper) + black pepper + basil (especially holy basil-thulasi) + garlic + lime juice + apple cider vinegar, will act *synergistically* in reducing hypertension, LDLC, sugar, obesity, diabetes and many chronic diseases. These herbs, in the order mentioned above, can be used in the ratio of, 4:2:1:1:2.5:1:1:2:1:1, respectively. Prepare** a mixture in the above ratio and consume about 5 to 10 g/day, along with or without honey/molasses/jiggery, depending on your other health problems, body weight, age etc. If you start this at early stages of these health problems, after 1 or 2 months, adjust the dose, depending on the results.

- **Watermelon seeds** contain an active principle, **cucurbocitrin;** it dilates blood vessels and reduces hypertension. Similarly, **curry leaves'** active principles, **murrayin & koenigin,** reduces hypertension and sugar.

- **Reduce salt/sodium in your diet.** One gram of salt supplies 400 mg of sodium; i.e. 40 % of salt is sodium. Persons having normal BP can limit dietary salt/sodium levels to not more than 5 g/2,000 mg (2 g) a day. However, those having high BP and senior people with greater salt sensitivity have to lower salt/sodium intake of 4 g/1,600 mg a day or less. Those who are having high blood pressure and those eating processed and further processed meats, high in sodium regularly, may take half the dose of salt, or less than 1500 mg of sodium/day. Those who are sweating heavily, like athletes, those doing heavy physical work, and those outside during hot sultry summers, the heavy sweating will lead to sodium loss. Hence, extra salt is needed to compensate this loss, up to 5 g/day. After 30 years of age, one must check their BP regularly and reduce the salt intake if the BP is high.

- Antioxidants, anti-stressors and nutraceuticals like vitamin-C & E, coenzyme-Q, mito-Q, will minimize the risk of CVD and other related diseases.

Non-dietary methods

As suggested in earlier chapters, **physical work and exercise** are the major steps to control blood sugar levels, diabetes, LDLC, TGL, CVD and obesity. Have a brisk walk for 30- 60 minutes daily plus yoga, meditation, breathing exercise, gym or stretching exercises for 30 minutes, depending on your age and other health problems. By proper diet management, as mentioned above, and exercise, all these chronic metabolic diseases can be kept under control with the least number of drugs, or even no drugs. However, blood glucose levels, serum lipid profiles and other tests must be checked, as per your doctors' advice, and must be followed. Do not stop medicines without your doctor's advice.

- Do special exercises to reduce body weight and waist size. Blood pressure often increases as weight and abdominal fat increases. Carrying too much weight around your waist can put you at greater risk of high blood pressure. Being overweight also can cause disrupted breathing while you sleep (sleep apnea), which further raises your blood pressure. Weight loss is one of the most effective lifestyle changes for controlling blood pressure. For waist size reduction, do special exercises, like waist twisting, as per the advice of a physiotherapist or a suitable trainer.

- Use blood thinners, like sustained release **aspirin,** at 1 mg/kg body weight, for free flow of blood in blood vessels and to prevent internal clotting.

- **Avoid all tobacco products**, including smoking, chewing, snuffing etc. which will narrow the blood vessels, leading to hypertension, >LDLC, and CVD.

- Maintaining correct body weight, BMI, keeping diabetes under control, preferably non-diabetic, consuming low calorie balanced diets rich in fiber, healthy food habits, walking, yoga, meditation, breathing exercise, swimming, other suitable exercises, active-positive-optimistic-disciplined lifestyle, minimizing mental stress, avoiding smoking and adequate sleep will supplement and compliment the medication if any, as per the doctor's advice, and will prevent, cure or keep CVD, LDLC, TGL, and hypertension under control.

Chapter 19

Dietary Methods to Control Cancer

Cancer, also called malignant tumor or neoplasms, is one of the top killer diseases in the world, with approximately 14 million new cases and 8.2 million cancer-related deaths in 2012. No country and no race is exempted from this catastrophe. Moreover, the incidences of cancer are increasing year after year. The number of new cases is expected to rise by about 70% over the next two decades. Among men, the most common sites of cancer diagnosed were lungs, prostate, large intestine, stomach and liver cancers. Among women the most common sites diagnosed were breast, large intestine, lungs, cervix and stomach cancers. More than 60% of the world's total new annual cases occur in Africa, Asia and Central and South America. These regions account for 70% of the world's cancer deaths. It is expected that annual cancer cases will rise from 14 million in 2012 to 22 million within the next two decades. The incidence of cancer rises dramatically with age, most likely due to a buildup of risks for specific cancers that increase with age.

Causes and predisposing factors for Cancer
Cancer is caused by some microbes, mostly viruses as well as due to chronic irritation/inflammation by many predisposing risk factors. The main viruses associated with human cancers are human papilloma virus, hepatitis B virus, hepatitis C virus, Epstein-Barr virus, human T-lymphotropic virus, Kaposi's sarcoma-associated herpes virus and Merkel cell polyoma virus. Besides viruses, bacteria like *Helicobacter pylori* causes ulcers and gasto-intestinal

cancer. Some internal parasites (helminthes), like *Clonorchis sinensis* and *Opisthorchis viverrini* also causes cancer.

HPV, HBV, HCV are responsible for up to 20% of cancer deaths in low- and middle-income countries. Infection with HIV – AIDS leads to immune-deficiency and substantially increases the risk of cancer, such as cervical cancer. Tobacco use, especially by smoking, is the most important risk factor for lung cancer, causing around 20% of global cancer deaths and around 70% of global lung cancer deaths. Some chronic infections like tuberculosis and ulcer are risk factors for cancer and have major relevance in low- and middle-income countries.

Non-dietary predisposing factors
Smoking, chronic alcoholism, high body mass index (obesity), lack of physical activity, behavioral changes, pollution of air, water, soil, food and surrounding environment, adulteration, microwaves, electronic gadgets, cell phones emitting several harmful rays and ultrasounds, automobile smoke, menstrual and menopause problems in women, prostate enlargement in men, sex with multiple partners, genetics, lack of immunity (disease resistance power), modern unhealthy sedentary lifestyle, mental stress of all kinds, especially emotional stress, drugs, drug misuse, cosmetics containing several chemicals, excess use of plastic in day-to-day life as containers for food and water, chemicals, and household chemicals are some of the non-dietary pre-disposing risk factors for cancer. In some cancer patients, excess radiotherapy itself causes many complications and death.

Carcinogens are chemicals and other toxic substances which predispose to cancer if exposed to a longer period, or at higher doses. Some of the carcinogens are asbestos, dioxins, benzene, gammaxene, formaldehyde, PVC, arsenic, lead, mercury, beryllium, cadmium, hexavalent-chromium, disinfectants, pesticides, herbi-cides, paints, keptone, factory emissions, especially from petro-chemical factories, coal mines, ethylene dioxide, all petroleum products, nickel, polyvinyl chloride, radium, ionizing and non-ionizing radiations, UV radiation, X-rays, gamma rays and other irradiations, detergents.

Dietary predisposing factors

Unhealthy food habits with low fiber foods, low fruit and vegetable intake, excess use of food chemicals, eating more junk foods and aerated soft drinks enriched with sugars and other chemicals, canned foods, refined foods, modified foods, highly processed and further processed foods, chronic constipation, cancer cells feeding foods like processed red meat, smoked meat, milk, irradiated foods, are some of the dietary predisposing risk factors, Even though they are not the direct causes of cancer, they may predispose the persons for more incidences of cancer if used in excess.

Cancer preventive measures

All the above may not cause cancer overnight; it may take decades. Moreover, they are cumulative and additive in nature. All those who have been exposed may not get cancer because of variations in their genetic makeup, disease resistance power, nutritional status, and other disease conditions, if any in them. Hence, to get rid of the potential for cancer, one must be aware of some of the avoidable causes, but we cannot avoid all the above causative agents (like pollution); we can only avoid as many of them as possible.

Non-dietary control measures

- More than 30% of cancer deaths could be prevented by modifying or avoiding the key risk factors mentioned above. Vaccinate against human papilloma virus (HPV), hepatitis B virus (HBV) and other cancer related diseases for which vaccines are available.

- Lack of sufficient fiber in the diet leads to constipation. Chronic constipation leads to diverticulitis (a condition where several small pouches are formed in the large intestine). Excretory material (stools) will accumulate in the diverticula, undergo fermentation and produce toxins. These toxins will lead to intestinal cancer as well as interfere with neuro-transmission, leading to autism and other neural disorders.

- Change to an active and positive lifestyle with more physical activities, like walking, exercise, yoga and meditation.

- Take preventive steps to avoid **occupational hazards**. Those who are working in chemical factories, coal mines, asbestos mines, petrochemical factories, tire manufacturing units, nuclear plants, X-ray and other radiation units in hospitals, must be extra cautious by taking proper steps like protective dress/apron, breathing unit, gloves, UV glasses etc. to avoid direct contact with hazardous chemicals, rays, fumes and smoke.

- Reduce exposure to non-ionizing radiation by sunlight (UV). Reduce exposure to ionizing radiation (occupational or medical diagnostic imaging).

- Minimize the use of chemicals at home like detergents, caustic soaps, cosmetics, bleaching powder, pesticides, fly repellants, insects control chemicals, garden chemicals etc. If using them, use safe products cautiously, without direct contact or exposure, following the instructions given by the manufacturer on the label.

- Do not use synthetic cosmetics, especially those having bleaching chemicals, lipsticks, skin creams made up of petroleum jelly, like Vaseline, soaps, shampoo, various sprays etc. which may cause skin cancer and maybe other types of cancers. Replace petroleum jelly with natural coconut oil, olive oil or butter oil (ghee). Natural herbal soaps and shampoos made up of soap nuts may be used.

- To the extent possible, replace hazardous chemicals with safe alternatives, like herbs and spices. As far as possible, try to live away from the pollution of all kinds, especially from automobiles and industries.

Dietary methods to control/prevent cancer

- If possible, drink fresh water from wells, springs, ponds, lakes etc. Preferably it may be heated to about 80° C (no boiling, only pasteurization just like milk) to kill the germs, but not to change the taste. Piped water and the so-called filter/mineral/bottled water in plastic bottles and cans may have some carcinogenic materials derived from the plastic containers and pipelines. During summer, drink water stored in earthenware (mud) pots. In USA and other developed countries, tap water is as safe as bottled water. To carry water to the office, school or during travel, use least reactive metal containers like stainless steel instead of plastic water bottles.

- Eat whole, unrefined, not further processed foods, such as whole grains, millets, pulses, beans, peas, lentils, without removing their skin. Preferably eat them after sprouting.

- Consume multiple fresh fruits, preferably all berries, guava, custard apple, apple, grapes, oranges, all melons, graviola and other seasonal foods, to the extent of 150 - 200 g /day. Avoid juices, jams, marmalades, tinned fruits etc.

- Consume fresh vegetables, especially those belonging to cruciferae family, like turnips, broccoli, cauliflower, cabbage, Brussels sprouts, & kale, beetroot, red carrot, all colour capsicums, radish, and all leafy vegetables, to the extent of 200-250 g/day.

- **Dietary fiber** prevents colon cancer and reduces cholesterol. So consume foods rich in fiber and low in calories, as mentioned in the earlier chapters. At least 25-40 g of soluble + insoluble fiber /day is needed to prevent all types of gastro-intestinal cancers, especially **colon cancer.**

- **National Cancer Institute of America (NCIA)** recommend-ded 25-35 g of fiber/day for cancer prevention and 30-40 g of fiber/day for body weight control. The fiber will swell in the intestine, help peristaltic bowel movement, prevent constipation, irritable bowel syndrome (IBS), diverticulitis, hemorrhoids (piles), binds with cholesterol in food and the bile and eliminates them from the body. On the other hand, excess fiber,>50 g /day, leads to indigestion and prevents absorption of some essential nutrients, especially zinc, iron, magnesium and many vitamins.

- **American Institute of Cancer Research (AICR)** suggests avoiding cancer cell feeding processed red meat and milk, and to consume plenty of fresh leafy vegetables and fruits, whole grains, germinated seeds, etc. and control weight gain.

- Do not cook or store foods in plastic containers. Use clay, earthenware, stainless steel and glass materials for cooking and storage of foods. Use stainless steel, earthen/clay pots and other non-reactive materials for cooking and storage.

- Recent research has proved that cooking in non-stick pans, coated with Teflon and other chemicals are carcinogenic and a health hazard. Hence, now these chemicals are replaced with safe, inactive enamel/china clay coating.

- Microwave and gas cooking may be substituted with electrical heaters and cookers.

- As far as possible consume homemade foods, prepared with whole grains, spices, pulses, vegetables and nuts, without adding preservatives, colors, flavors, nitrites, and other food additives. Avoid restaurant foods, especially sugary junk foods, aerated soft drinks, further processed foods, canned foods, irradiated foods, sweets, cookies, cakes, many sugar + salt + food colors + preservatives + food additives added foods.

- Sugar and sugar substitutes like aspartame and milk feed cancer cells. Hence avoid them.

- Cancer cells survive in an acid environment, like milk and red meat, but not in fish and chicken meat. Hence, avoid milk and red meat. Instead of cow's milk, take soya milk or rice milk.

- As reported in the herbs and spices chapter, **many herbs have anti-carcinogenic properties.** The active principle

curcumin in turmeric protects from **skin cancer** if applied topically, as turmeric cream. If consumed internally as a spice while preparing various dishes regularly, it will prevent various types of **gastrointestinal cancers.**

- **Graviola** or sour-sop fruit (native of Brazil) is from guyabano plant. Custard apple and *Rama phal* also belong to the same family. The guyabano/graviola/guanabana tree's fruits, leaves and seeds have **a powerful anti-cancer** principle called **graviolin, which is 10,000 times more powerful as an anti-cancer agent**. Many pharmaceutical companies have made futile attempts to synthesize and patent this graviolin. Many oncologists and local physicians in many countries are now using this plant's fruits, seeds and leaves for cancer treatment.

- Lycopene, a pigment as well as a powerful antioxidant present in tomato, red papaya, red guava, red pepper, beet-root, watermelon, red cabbage and red carrots has anti-carcinogenic , BP lowering and CVD controlling properties.

- Egg contains anti-carcinogenic pigments, Lumiflavin and Lumichrome, capable of preventing all forms of gastrointestinal cancers.

- Red coloured mushrooms, red reishi mushroom (Ganoderma lucidum) of Japan and lingzhi mushroom of China, also called medicinal mushrooms, have an anti-carcinogenic and immune-boosting active principle called lentinan, a poly-saccharide. It is available commercially in pharmacies as ganoderma extract. Regular consumption of this mushroom or this extract will reverse some types of cancer tissues into normal tissues.

- Herbs like Indian gooseberry (amla), Eclipta alba, Phylianthus neruri and turmeric are effective in preventing liver cancer, all types of hepatitis and jaundice.

- If cancer is detected early, regular use of ginseng (Ginseng panax), Aswagandha (Withania sominifera), turmeric, and green tea, Terminalia chebula, Arogya pacha (Trichopus zeylanicum) and/or Tinospora cardifolia, which possess anti-stress, immune-modulator and rejuvenator properties, will stimulate humoral and cell mediated immunity, cure AIDS and prevent several types of cancer.

- Nothapodytes foetida, an herb found in Western Ghats of India, contains camptothecin and has anti-carcinogenic properties. These capsules are already available in western market.

- All these herbs will act synergistically with modern allopathic anti-cancer drugs and boost their action. Herbs are safe and do not have any side effects. Moreover, they will reduce the side effects of radiation therapy and anti-cancer drugs.

Chapter 20

Dietary Tips to Control Arthritis, Autism and Eye Diseases

Arthritis management

At present arthritis, has become a common chronic disease, like diabetes and CVD. Previously only people above 60 years of age were having arthritis problems. Now it is common even in people below 30 years of age. There are different types of arthritis: osteoarthritis, rheumatoid arthritis, back pain, spondylitis, juvenile rheumatoid arthritis, osteoporosis, gout, bursitis, infectious arthritis etc. Of these, osteoarthritis and rheumatoid arthritis are more common. Osteoarthritis is age related, mostly seen in elderly people, due to wear and tear of joints and bones or to an injury. Whereas, rheumatoid arthritis and juvenile rheumatoid arthritis are also seen in younger people, and is considered as autoimmune diseases, which means the body's immune system turns on itself and attacks the joints. Hence, the treatment, management and dietary plans differ for different types of arthritis. For all types of arthritis, avoid exposure to cold, take hot water baths, do not take cool drinks, and **do exercises** recommended by an orthopedician or physiotherapist.

Foods suitable for arthritis, especially rheumatoid arthritis patients, are n-3 PUFA (omega-3 fatty acids) rich foods like fish, flax seeds, horse gram, chia seeds, beetroot, carrot, cinnamon, ginger, garlic, turmeric, basil, thyme, cloves, cardamom, red pepper, black pepper, orange, strawberry and vitamins-A, D& E. American College of Rheumatology and Arthritis Foundation of America recommends anti-inflammatory foods, spices and herbs suitable for arthritis patients. Some of them are olive oil, grape seed oil, avocado oil, sesame oil, coconut oil, capsicum, dill, fish, peas, ginger, broccoli, vitamin-D, cranberries, boswellic acid, *Euonymus alatus* (Devil's claw) and *Triptergium wilfordii* (Thunder God vine).

Foods and food supplements suitable for osteoarthritis patients are fish, n-3 PUFA, prawns, crab, lobster, calcium, phosphorus, magnesium, vitamin-D3, Hy-D, glucosamine, chondroitin sulphate, methyl-sulfonyl-methane (MSM), hyaluronic acid and most of the foods suggested above. Recommended exercises, yoga and physiotherapy are also equally important to keep arthritis under control.

As per American College of Rheumatology, the **foods *not suitable* for arthritis** patients are gluten rich foods like wheat and barley, dairy products, corn, potato, tapioca, red meat, sugar, salt, coffee, tomato, certain nuts like peanuts, omega-6 rich oils like sunflower, corn, soya and safflower oils, eggplant (brinjal), alcohol, refined CHO rich foods like cookies, pastries, bagels, muffins, cakes, chocolates, French fries and chips.

Herbs, ***vetiveria zizanioides*** (an aromatic hairy grass roots), ***Cardiospermum helicacaban*** (used as a fruit and vegetable), *Euonymus alatus* (Devil's claw) and *Triptergium wilfordii* (Thunder God vine) are used in Ayurveda as herbal medicines for relieving rheumatism, stiffness of joints and sprains.

Autism control
Autism is a neuro-biological pervasive developmental spectrum disorder noticed in young children, which may gradually disappear as they grow older. Incidences of autism have increased nearly 50-fold over the last 40 years. Now one in 100 children born has autism. Such children will have deficiency in developmental, social, behavioral, communication skills and eye contact. The degree of symptoms varies with individuals. Early detection and care will

suppress the symptoms, and they recover quickly in a few years. If proper care is taken autism can be prevented and cured at an early age. Even though there is no authenticated treatment for autism in modern allopathic medicine, certain herbs, spices and foods, along with multi-vitamin, minerals, amino acid and omega-3 supplementation, gastro-intestinal cleaning/corrective measures, neural toning, QST (Qigong Sensory Treatment) message, occupational therapy and exercise are natural treatments.

Just like other chronic diseases, pollution of various kinds, unhealthy modern lifestyle, especially excess eating of **junk foods** having several **food additives, chemicals, pesticides, herbicides, sugar, refined starch** (Maida/bakers' flour), lack of sufficient fiber fruits, vegetables and greens in the diet, nicotine, caffeine, alcohol, toxins of various kinds, will predispose the children to autism. Autism children will invariably have digestive disorders, unclean gut, chronic constipation, insufficient sleep and exercise, which will aggravate the symptoms. Hence, they have to be avoided to get rid of autism. Children born to mothers having the above described lifestyle and food habits have more chances to have autism at birth.

Since autism is mainly seen in children, once they enter the teen age, they can take these foods, gradually. But it is better to avoid junk foods, rich in food additives, refined starch and sugar, because they will predispose the persons to other chronic diseases like diabetes, obesity, cardio-vascular diseases, cancer, arthritis etc.

Diet & other tips to control autism

- Autism persons must consume gluten-free, casein-free, harmful food additives-free, soya-free (can take soya foods, if they take multi-enzyme capsules having phytase enzyme) and sugar-free foods.

- Eat unprocessed/least processed wholesome foods, prepared at home.

- Eat **omega-3 fatty acids** (n-3) rich foods, like **fish** (wild Alaskan salmon preferred), flax seeds, chia seeds, walnuts or n-3 fish oil + **krill oil** capsules @ pediatric dose.

- Eat essential amino acid **tryptophan** rich foods like turkey meat, eggs, chicken, fish and lean red meat also. If necessary **5-hydroxy tryptophan (5-HTP) capsules** can be consumed @ ½ to 1 g/day, depending on the age of the child. It is the precursor for the synthesis of the neurotransmitter **serotonin,** also called as **happiness factor**. If necessary, serotonin capsules may be consumed regularly.

- Similarly, another neurotransmitter, gamma amino butyric acid (GABA) capsules, which are available in the market, may be consumed alternatively.

- Take **bone soup or broth**, with added pepper and turmeric, to supply essential nutrients and immune-modulators.

- Take foods rich in **probiotics**, like fermented foods such as **yoghurt, buttermilk, curd,** kefir, amasai, sauerkraut or kimchi. Alternatively, take **probiotic gummies** or capsules @ pediatric dose.

- Consuming **digestive multi-enzymes capsules,** containing the enzyme, **phytase,** after each meal is recommended to avoid digestive problems and leaky gut.

- The symptoms of autism can be reduced by vitamin B6, B12, vitamin A, C & D, folate, omega-3 fatty acids, magnesium, zinc, manganese and organic selenium. Hence, supplementation of multi-mineral + vitamins supplements at pediatric dose is good to overcome autism for healthy brain function and strong bones.

- Drink plenty of clean, un-fluoridated water, at least eight glasses of reverse osmosis water a day.

- Amino acid L-carnitine, 250-500 mg daily, has been shown to reduce the symptoms of autism.

- Other amino acid derivatives, liposomal glutathione and l-glutamine supplementation, if available in the market, can be given, as per the specifications on the label.

- Fresh green leafy vegetables supplementation daily will relive from autism.

- Fresh fruits, rich in potassium, magnesium have to be consumed daily.

What not to eat

- Avoid all gluten rich foods made with wheat, maida (bakers' flour/refined flour), barley and rye, such as bread and all bakery products (except oats bread), pasta, noodles etc.

- **Cow's milk** and other dairy products contain a protein called **A1 casein,** which can trigger a similar reaction as gluten, and therefore, should be avoided. However, milk from zebu cow (cattle having the hump), buffalo, goat, camel, donkey, horse is free from this A-1 casein. Hence, they can be consumed, if available.

- Sugar can cause fluctuation in blood sugar level, leading to behavioral problems. Avoid any forms of sugar, especially artificial soft drinks (sodas), fruit juices, candy, desserts, cakes, ice creams, sweets, etc.

- Also, avoid sugar substitutes like aspartame, food colors, flavors, preservatives and other food additives.

- Soya products contain phytic acid which can irritate the intestines causing leaky gut. However, soya products can be consumed if an enzyme supplement containing phytase enzyme is taken daily. Isolated soy protein, free from phytic acid can be consumed.

Herbs & spices which will bring positive changes and control autism

- There are several herbs used in Ayurveda for autism control: essential oils from vetiver oil, from *Vetiveria zizanioides* plant (a grass grown in tropical sandy soils), lavender oil, cinnamaldehyde (from cinnamon), carvacrol (from oregano), thyme oil, clove oil, nutmeg oil, peppermint oil, frankincense oil, *Piper longum* (long pepper/tail pepper), lemon balm (*Meliesa officinalis*) etc. have proven to balance the brain waves, calm the body and support neurological development, which will support natural autism treatments.

- *Cardiospermum helicacaban* (tomatillo) is a creeper, with its fruits resembling like small tomato inside a leafy cover. **Tomatillo** will act as a natural laxative, neutralizes toxins and cure nervous disorders.

- Ashwagandha (*Withania Somneifera*) shows high affinity for GABA (gamma amino butyric acid) receptors, which can be used in the treatment of memory loss, anxiety, attention deficit etc. which are common features of autism.

- Another herb, *Griffonia simplicifolia,* is a rich source of **5-hydroxy tryptophan (5-HTP),** and is a good neurotransmitter, like serotonin and GABA, which can reduce the severity of autism.

- **Shankhapushpi or conch flower (*Clitoria ternatia*), a climber plant, especially its roots,** increases the acetylcholine (ACh) content in the brain, the neurochemical basis for improvised learning and memory.

- Brahmi (*Bacopa monneiri)* and shatavari (*Asperagus racemosus)* are considered as brain tonics, which will increase the memory, improve the focus and relieve anxiety. It is available in tablets form in India, USA and other countries.

- Swarna pathri (*Cassia augustifolia*) is a safe and effective herb to prevent constipation, clean up the digestive system and stimulate the nervous system indirectly. It is available in tablets form in India, USA and other countries.

- More effective home remedy to control autism will be: take a mixture of brahmi: Swarna pathri: Shanku pushpi: karakkai (*picrorhiza kurroa*); aswagandha or ginseng : turmeric powder: ginger: *Cardiospermum helicacaban* : pepper : lemon balm herbs :: 4:4:2:4:2:2:2:2;1:1 ratio. Mix them in the above ratio and take 5-10 g/day, depending on the age, mixed with 2-3 ml of lime juice, 2 ml apple cider vinegar and 1 spoon honey at the morning before breakfast. Within one month significant improvement will be noticed.

Non-dietary supportive measures

- **Avoid constipation**. This is the most essential step to overcome autism, diverticulitis and colon cancer. During constipation, part of the undigested food will not come out as stool and will get accumulated in the large intestine in the several diverticula (small pouches) formed. There, the stools will undergo bacterial decomposition, releasing several toxins, which will interfere with neurotransmitter mechanism, causing autism and other neurological disorders. Moreover, these toxins and diverticulitis will lead to colon cancer. Therefore, keep regular bowel evacuation daily, preferably twice a day. If you need support, magnesium sulphate (at lower dose 5-10 g, once a week) safe herbal laxatives preparations like swarna pathri, aloe vera, senna are good laxatives for gut cleaning. Pure **castor oil,** 10 to 30 ml may be taken in the morning on an empty stomach, as a purgative, to cleanse the gut once a month.

- One of the most closely related symptoms/conditions to autism is poor sleep habits, which may be due to **insufficient melatonin production. Melatonin is a sleep hormone produced by the pineal gland in the brain, which induces sound sleep, reduces stress, relaxes the brain and thereby alleviates autism.** Certain herbs and spices like turmeric, ashwagandha, ***Rhodiola rosea*, Saint John's wort** and chamomile flowers, will boost melatonin production. Serotonin, produced in the body, also boosts melatonin production and induces sleep. Melatonin is a natural, safe product, with no side effects, and is available in pharmacies in various strengths; 0.5 to 1 mg strength is sufficient for children.

- Serotonin, also called happiness factor, is a motivation neurotransmitter that plays a large role in mood, learning, appetite control and sleep. Serotonin keeps people more relaxed, calm, worries don't seem as big, anxiety disappears, reduces insomnia and digestive disorders and used by millions to relieve symptoms of depression. Several serotonin supplements to restore serotonin deficiency are available in the market.

- GABA (gamma amino butyric acid) is another neurotransmitter, producing similar results like serotonin, and has been clinically proven to boost GABA and serotonin levels in human body.

- Take serotonin and GABA boosting supplements like tryptophan, turmeric + black pepper, B-complex, N-3 PUFA, 5-HTP, L-Theanine, Cartigon, dopamine, acetylcholine, SAMe (S-adenosyl methionine), ashwagandha, passion flower, lemon balm, Saint John's Wort, Rhodiola rosea are good boosters. Exercise, sleep and sunlight boost serotonin secretion. Another hormone, melatonin, is secreted by the pineal gland in the brain. It is a sleep hormone, and it induces sound sleep without any side effects.

- QST (Qigong Sensory Treatment) massaging or rubbing of fingers and cheeks of the child in the morning before bath may help support muscle strength needed for speech and chewing. It also improves the neurotransmission and brain functioning.

- Detox baths using magnesium sulphate in hot water once a week is recommended.

- Exercise or find another way to sweat profusely at least three times a week. You could try using a sauna, steam or detox bath along with exercise. Do relaxation exercises every day to get the nervous system in a state of calm and relaxed.

- Take the advice of an occupational therapist, periodically.

Dietary methods to control eye diseases

Among the diseases of the eyes, cataract, glaucoma, night blindness, diabetic retinopathy (DR), macular degeneration (MD) and retinitis pigmentosa (RP) are common, which can be prevented, or the intensity can be reduced, by proper dietary and non-dietary management. The last three diseases affect the retina of the eyes, resulting in partial or total loss of vision, reduced night vision and/or narrow tubular vision. Cataract and glaucoma can be delayed or prevented by protecting eyes from direct sunlight/UV rays, dust, fumes and gases and other radiation/chemical hazards. Glaucoma is sometimes associated with hypertension. Supplementation of vitamin-A or its precursors, the carotenoid pigments, also delays occurrence of these diseases. Simple night blindness, which is due to vitamin-A deficiency, can be corrected by supplementation of vitamin-A or its precursors.

However, DR, MD and RP are complicated retinal diseases. MD is mostly an age-related disease, and incidences are higher in diabetic patients. Retinopathy is another retinal disease seen in advanced cases of diabetes, with uncontrollable blood sugar levels. In both these diseases, the retina may get detached, undergoes degeneration and photoreceptors, rods and cones will get atrophied, resulting in loss of blood supply and loss of vision. If proper care is taken at the early stages of onset, the vision can be partially restored.

RP is a genetic disorder, caused due to several gene aberrations in both autosomal and sex-linked genes, both dominant and recessive.

It is even seen in children born to normal non-carrier parents, not having any family history, due to mutation of genes. Changes in the environment, pollution of various kinds, chemicals like formaldehyde, radiation, junk foods and refined foods having several mutagenic chemicals, are responsible for these mutations and chromosomal aberrations. Children born to parents who are closely related have higher chances of getting the RP.

In RP patients, the rods and cones, the photoreceptors in the retina, undergo degeneration, gradual reduction in the field of vision and finally resulting in tubular vision and even loss of eyesight, depending on the genes involved and the care taken by the patients. Even though there is no proven treatment for RP, supplementation of vitamin-A palmitate (not acetate) and a few supportive herbals suggested below will reduce the progression of the RP. Stem cell therapy and special eye spectacles are still under research.

Herbs, spices & foods to improve eyesight

1. All fresh fruits, especially, wild berries like bilberry, huckleberry, blueberry, blackberry, maqui berry, Indian blackberry, red guava, citrus fruits, apricot, plumes, prunes, red grapes, red papaya, avocado, watermelon, strawberry, mangos etc. are good for eyes.

2. All fresh vegetables, especially red chili, red/orange bell pepper/capsicum, tomato, red cabbage, broccoli, beetroot, sweet potato, red/orange carrot, asparagus, Brussel sprouts, red cauliflower, red radish, etc. will have pigments lutein, luteolin, kryptoxanthin, zeaxanthin and other carotinoid pigments, which will nourish the retina.

3. All fresh leafy vegetables like kale, spinach, *Eclypta* family (ponnaganti leaves) drumstick leaves, alfalfa (lucern), parsley, mint, curry leaves, coriander leaves (cilantro), red lettuce, dandelion and any red leafy vegetables are good for retinal health.

4. **Spices:** Turmeric (curcumin), black pepper, red pepper/ paprika powder, cayenne pepper (long variety of red pepper), rosemary and basil.

5. **Herbs**: Gingko biloba, holy basil (tulasi) or ordinary basil, milk thistle, *Eclypta alba* (bringaraj).

6. **Vitamins and minerals:** vitamin-A palmitate (not acetate) = 10,000 to 15,000 I.U./day, inositol (B-8 vitamin), copper and zinc.

7. **Others:** Carotenoid pigments (beta-carotene, cryptoxanthin, **lutein**, zeaxanthin, lycopene), **omega-3 fatty acids, especially DHA,** pumpkin seeds, egg yolks, buck wheat (you can use it to make upma, pongal, gruel and as rice substitutes), L-Lysine (an essential amino acid), hemp seeds, walnuts, anti-oxidants present in all fresh fruits and vegetables, blood thinner like Asperin-81 (1 tab daily), which will allow free flow of blood into retina.

8. **Non-dietary methods**

- Avoid (or keep them under control) diabetes, obesity, hypertension and other predisposing diseases.

- Do regular exercise, walking, yoga (including Sirshasanam - upside down) and meditation for one hour a day. Do deep breathing exercises, have positive thinking, be cheerful, optimistic and calm.

- Use UV protective glasses while walking in bright sun light.

- Do exercise to eyes like, eyeballs rotation, up and down, left to right and rotation movements, for about 3-5 minutes twice daily.

9. **Things to AVOID:** vitamin-E, all mental stress, including emotional stress & **stress to eyes** due to bright light, UV rays, over exposure to electronic light from TV, computers etc. (not avoidable?)

Practical methods

1. Consume as much as possible **turmeric powder** (need not be costly curcumin) through regular foods as well as additional supplementation. Use turmeric powder liberally in all foods you eat. It is not only good for RP, but it will boost general immunity and prevent many diseases like cancer, skin infections, flu, sore throat, intestinal disorders, nervous disorders.

2. Black pepper will boost the action of turmeric. So prepare a mixture of 90% turmeric + 10% black pepper and consume ½ teaspoon (about 2 g) twice daily in the morning and night. At night, add this mixture to a glass of hot milk and drink after supper, half an hour before bedtime. This will also give you good sleep. This is in addition to the turmeric in regular foods.

3. Take 1 g of fish/krill oil capsule daily for omega-3 fatty acids.

4. Take 1 lutein capsules daily or prepare a mixture of deep orange marigold flower petals + red pepper/ chili powder in equal quantities & consume ½ teaspoon, twice daily.

5. Swallow one vitamin-A palmitate = 10,000-15,000 IU (Aquasol-A or Palmitate-A) daily.

6. Consume **fresh leafy vegetables & other vegetables** mentioned above liberally, to the extent of 250- to 300 g of mixed vegetables/salads (preferably, avoid salad dressings)/day & **fresh mixed fruits** mentioned above @ 200-250 g/day.

7. Use herbs and spices mentioned above to the extent possible and available.

8. Eat 10-15 g of mixed nuts like walnuts, pumpkin seeds, flax, chia seeds daily.

Chapter 21

Dietary Tips for Healthy Living

In the earlier chapters, several dietary and non-dietary guidelines were given to overcome several health-related problems, especially chronic metabolic diseases and disorders like CVD, hypertension, >LDLC, >TGL, obesity, diabetes and cancer. Nutrition and an active-healthy lifestyle plays a greater role in disease prevention and control, sometimes more than the medicines. Balanced, wholesome foods, along with an active, healthy lifestyle boosts immunity, i.e. increases the disease resistance power and thereby prevents the basic occurrence of any disease. If a disease does strike, it will be mild and will subside quickly. Nutrition also optimizes the immunity development due to vaccination. Hence, much attention must be placed on consuming balanced wholesome foods and leading an active, healthy lifestyle. The dietary guidelines given in the earlier chapters are summed up here, with some additional information. For more details, refer to previous chapters.

Dietary guidelines for healthy living

- Eat foods made up of **whole grains. Multi-grains** are preferred rather than a single grain. Avoid polished and refined grains, which are mostly made up of diabeto-genic, high glycemic index starch, with very little or no fiber. **Brown rice and brown bread** is better than white rice/bread. All **millets, sorghum, quinoa, oats, barley, rye, buckwheat, wild rice, triticale and ancient minor grains** are nutritionally superior grains than traditional, high-energy corn, wheat and rice. Diabetes, obesity and CVD will not come near persons eating these minor grains on a regular basis.

- As protein source, especially for vegetarians and vegans, consume multiple varieties of **whole beans, legumes, lentils, nuts, peas** and **pulses,** without removing their outer skin, which is rich in fiber, minerals and vitamins. Sprouting them and eating the sprouts will be a better way of consuming them.

- **In a healthy diet the ideal proportions of multi-grains: beans/pulses (vegetable protein sources): mixed vegetables: fruits: milk: and other animal proteins (eggs + chicken + fish), must be in the ratio of 30: 15: 20: 15: 10: 10. This is equivalent to 30%, multiple whole grains, 15% multiple beans/pulses and nuts, 20% mixed vegetables, including green leafy vegetables, 15% mixed fruits, 10% milk and 10% meats (eggs + meat). For vegetarians, the meat portion should be substituted with beans, nuts and pulses, on equal protein basis.**

- **For obese and diabetic persons, the above ratios must be 25% grains, 15% vegetable protein sources, 23% mixed vetables, 15% mixed fruits, 10% milk products and 12 % animal protein sources (egg +fish + chicken.**

- Eat fruits separately. Do not combine fruits with regular meals because it will cause fermentation and other complications. Eat mixed fruits instead of snacks, either between breakfast and lunch or at tea time in the evening.

- Eat **fresh fruits** as whole instead of fruit juices, jams, marmalades and canned fruits. Even the so-called smoothies and fruit juices in cans and restaurants are having added sugars, colors and preservatives, which are not good for health.

- **Wash fruits and vegetables, especially leafy vegetables**, with running water before cooking or eating to remove dirt, pesticides, wax and other harmful chemicals used for their preservation. In case of organic foods, wash to a lesser extent, because they are free from pesticide residues, but they will have dirt and other contaminants from handling and transporting.

- Do not peel the skin of apples, peaches, plums, tomatoes, grapes, nectarines and the inner thin white skins of oranges and other citrus fruits. Do not discard the seeds of grapes, guava etc. because they are rich in fiber and many health promoting active principles, as reported in Table-13-1. Even the inner white portion of certain bananas' skin is rich in fiber, and reduces kidney and gallstones. Hence, scrap and eat it.

- Eat **150 to 250 g of fresh mixed vegetables,** which includes 50-100 g of fresh green leafy vegetables. Some vegetables like cucumber, lettuce, carrot and beetroot can be eaten raw, after washing. Avoid canned vegetables.

- Different **beans, legumes, lentils, nuts, peas and pulses** form part of a healthy diet as protein supplement; especially for vegetarians. The quantity varies from 20-50 g/day, depending on the non-vegetarian foods you are consuming. You can take many of them as evening snacks, replacing junk foods. Eat fried (not deep fried) or boiled peas, chickpea, pigeon pea, green lentil, different beans, horse gram, mung beans, peanuts, flax, chia, walnuts, cashews, almonds and other nuts, depending on your budget and local availability.

- **Milk** is good for all, except for cancer patients and those having allergies for lactose and casein, because it will feed the cancer cells. Nutritionally and medicinally, goat milk is better than cow's milk. Camel milk is equally good. In some Asian countries and in Europe donkey milk is getting popular due to its health promoting properties, and is sold at a premium price. Buffalo milk, due to its high fat content (8-9%), may not be suitable to consume as it is, except for athletes, growing children and lean persons (<20 BMI), but can be consumed after fat reduction to 2-4%. Similarly, 4%

fat whole cow's milk is good for all, except for seniors above 60 years and those having high triglycerides (TGL), who can take 2% fat milk. Skim milk is not so good. Daily 300-500 ml of 2-4% milk can be consumed.

- Consuming one glass of hot milk, mixed with ½ teaspoon (2-3 g) of turmeric powder + 1 g of black pepper, half to one hour before bed, promotes sound sleep as well as boosting immunity and reducing blood pressure.

- **Eggs** are excellent food for all, especially for growing children, athletes, pregnant and lactating women, convalescents, weak persons, seniors, diabetics, obese, cancer, arthritis patients. It has the highest biological value and immune boosting properties. Hence, all can consume one or two eggs daily. Now in developed countries, the USA, Europe, Japan and China, for dieting purpose and convenience, people are taking two eggs for breakfast. It is a satiety food, so they can skip lunch and reduce body weight. Scientifically, it has been proven beyond doubt that egg cholesterol (even any food cholesterol) has no correlation with serum cholesterol. Based on several strong scientific evidences, the ADA, AHA, USDA and authorities in many other countries have removed earlier restrictions on cholesterol consumption. WHO is also recommending a minimum of half egg/day, and there is no upper limit. Unfortunately, in India the egg consumption is very low at <60 eggs/annum, due to several unscientific misconceptions, beliefs and negative propaganda, which is one of the lowest egg consumption in the world. Table egg does not have any life. It is the only unadulterated whole food on earth. For more details refer to Chapters One, Seven, Eight and Nine.

- Drink two to three liters of **water** per day, depending on the water content in the foods, weather/season, sweating and exercise. Take more water after getting up from bed in the morning and after physical exercise. Take less water during eating and during nights. Take water if you are thirsty. For more details, refer to Chapter Four on water requirement.

- **Fish** is an excellent food, rich in high quality protein and omega-3 fatty acids (n-3 PUFA). For good health, people can consume 50-100 g or more fish daily. Do not remove the skin of fish, because it is the source of the n-3 PUFA.

- **Chicken** meat is considered a white meat, like fish. Tender broiler chicken meat, without skin, will have low 3-5 % fat and negligible cholesterol, with good levels of healthy MUFA, like olive oil. In India, the chicken consumption is in the bottom of the world, with just 2.3 kg/annum, whereas, in many countries it is more than 50 kg. Hence, to prevent protein deficiency at least 50 g of broiler meat/day (18.25 kg /annum) should be consumed, along with other protein sources.

- **Diabetics** should reduce the meal size and have small snacks in between meals. They must take foods rich in complex CHO, proteins and lipids, and avoid simple sugars and refined CHO. The energy for a diabetic must come from complex CHO=50%, lipids=33% and proteins=17%. **The total energy must not exceed the recommended calories, as suggested in the earlier chapters**. If they are overweight, they must restrict calories also.

- If you want to eat sweets, ice cream, cakes etc., eat them occasionally, but proportionally cut calories from other sources so that the total calorie intake will not exceed the recommended levels. Sugar-free sweets, using sugar substitutes, are equally bad or even worse, because many of them are carcinogenic.

- **Sugar** and sugar substitutes are the worst foods and are enemies of mankind, because sugar is more habit forming than heroin and predisposes us to so many diseases. It is not an essential nutrient, not needed in the diet, no RDA for it; it supplies only empty calories. So, keep away from sugars and all sugar-containing foods. Sugar is even harmful for teeth and mouth, whereas, **salt,** another harmful food, is good for teeth and mouth for gargling purpose.

- **Avoid all junk foods** like sweets, cookies, cakes, ice creams, French fries, chips, pastries sodas, artificial sweet drinks, refined foods, burgers, pastas, pizzas made up of refined flour, sugar, trans-fatty acids, butter, ghee, hydrogenated fat having only calorific value (empty calorie foods) and various **harmful food additives**, like flavoring agents, preservatives, conditioners, binders, pigments etc., as described in earlier chapters. **Avoid all foods having many food additives, especially avoid soft drinks and sodas.**

- As far as possible **eat homemade foods,** free from food additives and avoid restaurant foods (from street foods to seven-star hotel foods), because they will add several food additives, described in Chapter Eleven on food additives, to enhance eye appeal, flavor, crispiness and eating qualities of their foods. As Dr. Lundell said, eat **"homemade, grandma foods,"** having no food additives, similar to foods prepared earlier to 1950.

- **Vitamins and mineral supplements are optional.** If you eat a well-balanced diet, there is no need for any vitamins and mineral supplementation. Do not take any minerals or vitamins at therapeutic dose or RDA regularly, because your food will supply many of them, and it may damage your liver and other vital organs. Take slightly lesser than the RDA or preventive dose. Therapeutic doses are needed only under disease conditions, pregnancy and during breast feeding period, under a doctor's supervision. Obese persons, who are restricting the food intake, shall take vitamin and mineral supplements, regularly.

- **Probiotics** are beneficial symbiotic microbes, harboring or colonizing in our gastro-intestinal tract, especially in the large intestine. The common probiotic microbes belong to *Lactobacillus, Bifidobacterium, Saccharomyces (yeast)* and

Streptococcus species. The main purpose of probiotics is to prevent colonization of harmful microbes like salmonella in the intestine, which will cause several infections. The main sources of probiotics in our foods are yoghurt, curd, buttermilk and many other fermentation products. Now probiotic capsules are available in the pharmacies. There is no need to consume probiotic capsules regularly; instead, take probiotic foods, as mentioned above. However, when you take antibiotics orally to treat some infectious disease, some of the probiotics may be destroyed. Hence, in such case i.e. post-antibiotic treatment, you can take probiotic capsules to replace the lost ones.

Food habits

- Besides foods, food habits are equally important for better health. Food habits include timely eating of meals, split feeding, no overeating, do not drink much water during eating, eating balanced foods, do not eat too hot or too cold foods, eat slowly by enjoying the food and do not skip any meal, especially breakfast.

- Eat food in a calm and pleasant atmosphere, preferably sharing with family members and friends. Chew the food well before swallowing.

- Gargle your mouth, preferably with hot water, after each food, including drinks, to remove food particles in the mouth and in between teeth. If not properly removed, they will undergo bacterial fermentation, leading to teeth and gum decay and several other health problems.

- In case of throat infection (sore throat), gargle the mouth with hot water containing salt and turmeric powder, especially after supper.

- Salt is good for teeth, but bad for heart, whereas, sugar is bad for all parts of the body.

- Eat food moderately and never eat until completely full. Eat to three-fourths stomach full, never until a full stomach. Split daily food to more than 4 times a day, preferably 5 or 6 times, instead of 2-3 heavy meals. The total food intake per day shall not exceed the dietary calories and other nutrients recommended for a day (RDA). Have small meals at frequent intervals. This is especially essential for diabetic patients. If you are not hungry, skip one meal or take a liquid diet, like buttermilk, coconut water, or take some fruits and salads instead of regular food.

- **Appropriate eating schedule:** 5-6 am = 1 cup of milk /tea or coffee, without sugar; 7-8 am = breakfast; 10-11 am = whole fruit mixture, about 200 g; 1-2 pm = lunch; 4-5 pm = mixed vegetables + sprouted grains salads, preferably without any salad dressing (or sugar-free salad dressing); 7-8 pm = dinner; 9 pm = 1 cup of 2% fat milk without sugar, but add ½ teaspoon turmeric powder. Diabetics can snack in between, but the total calories shall not exceed those prescribed.

- Take a hearty breakfast like a prince, eat light lunch like a poor man, and eat dinner moderately like a common man. Eat enough hearty breakfast, with satiety foods like eggs, cheese, soya protein or meats, which will suppress hunger. Take a light lunch containing sprouted grains, fruits, curd, buttermilk, yogurt and vegetable salads. Have a moderate supper with whole grains, salads, soup etc.

- **Both fasting and feasting are not good for health**. However, fasting is good during high fever, stomach upset, indigestion, vomiting, anorexia (lack of appetite), jaundice and many other gastro-intestinal disorders.

- **Fasting for weight reduction purpose will not be effective.** Sometimes it may have negative results. Frequent fasting for religious purpose is also not good.

- **Feasting** is not at all good under any circumstances. However, if you have to take a feast during marriages etc., eat moderately or skip next one or two meals.

- Do not skip any meal, especially breakfast. At the same time, do not over eat. If you are not hungry, skip a meal. If this non-appetite is a chronic problem, take the doctors' advice.

- Check body weight at least once a month and adjust food accordingly. Maintain normal body weight and body mass index, between 20 - 24. Reduce waistline, because abdominal fat is more dangerous for heart, raises BP and causes difficulty in breathing (dyspnea).

- It may be difficult even for well-educated persons to know whether they are taking the correct calories they need. The simple rule is, if a person is consuming the correct calories they need, men over 25 years and women over 20 years of age (except during pregnancy and breast feeding) shall not gain or lose any body weight, because such weight gain after this age is nothing but body fat. Moreover, they must maintain correct body mass index (BMI) of 20-24. Calculation of BMI and daily energy requirements are shown in Chapter Sixteen. So, measure your body weight at least once a month and plan your diet accordingly.

- There are several reasons for overweight and obesity. Diet alone may not be the reason. Family history, hypothyroidism, irregular menstrual cycle in women, corticosteroid drugs, anabolic steroid drugs, sedentary habits and a combination of these factors may influence obesity. Hence, overweight persons should take the advice of a qualified physician, to trace the reason and rectify the defect. For details on obesity, refer Chapter Sixteen on obesity.

Non-dietary tips for healthy living

- **Constipation** is the prime cause for several chronic diseases. Eating refined sugary junk foods, with no/least fiber will cause constipation. If there is no regular daily bowel evacuation, the stools will accumulate in the large intestine, by forming several small pouches like diverticula, called **diverticulitis**. Here the stools will undergo bacterial decomposition, producing several toxins, which in turn produce several diseases, interfere with neurotransmission, suppress immunity and cause colon cancer. Hence, constipation must be prevented at any cost by taking fiber rich foods, especially leafy vegetables regularly. If necessary, take laxatives, preferably herbals like *Swarna pathri*, as mentioned in herbal chapter, earlier. Once a month take a purgative like castor oil or magnesium sulphate to clean the gut.

- Do not sleep soon after eating. There must be two to three hour's gap, preferably three hours, between supper and going to bed. Eat supper at 7 p.m. and go to bed at 10 p.m.

- Have sufficient sleep. Children must sleep for 8-10 hours, depending on the age. Adults must sleep for about 7 hours a day and seniors for 8 hours/day. Insufficient sleep leads to several neurological and psychological disorders. Avoid coffee during nights. In case of sleep apnea, consult a doctor or take **melatonin** tablets, which is a normal sleep hormone produced by the pineal endocrine gland, within the brain.

- Do not sleep during daytime. But senior citizens, patients, pregnant and lactating women and children below 10 years can sleep for an hour or two after lunch. Babies and very young children also need more sleeping hours, ranging from 10-20 hours.

- **Exercise and other physical activities** are a must for a healthy body and weight maintenance. Depending on your age and time, do walking, jogging, cycling, yoga, meditation, gardening, swimming, aerobic exercises, playing active games which need physical work and going to a gym, in addition to routine household and office work. One must do some sort of physical exercise for half to one hour daily, depending on their age and other conditions.

- **Avoid smoking totally**. It is the primary cause for many diseases of heart, lungs and other organs. Even the breathing of smoke from smokers is harmful for health. Hence, avoid mixing with smokers when they are smoking.

- **Do not become an alcoholic**. If you are using alcohol, drink to moderation, not more than 24 ml of pure alcohol (based on the alcohol content in the drink) per day for men and 12 ml for women. Pregnant and breast feeding mothers shall not drink. Among the drinks, red wine is a better drink due to its good HDLC enhancing property. Alcohol supplies 7 calories per gram. Since alcohol is habit forming and involves extra expenditure, **it is better and safer to avoid alcohol. Keep away from drugs also.**

- Have positive thoughts, be optimistic, develop friendships and family relationships well and spend some time with them. Go out frequently with family members or friends for relaxation. Do not remain lonely; get rid of negative ideas, evils, stress, greediness, tension and depression. Develop a good hobby like book reading, social service, games, sports, pilgrimage, travel etc., which will occupy you actively and positively.

Index

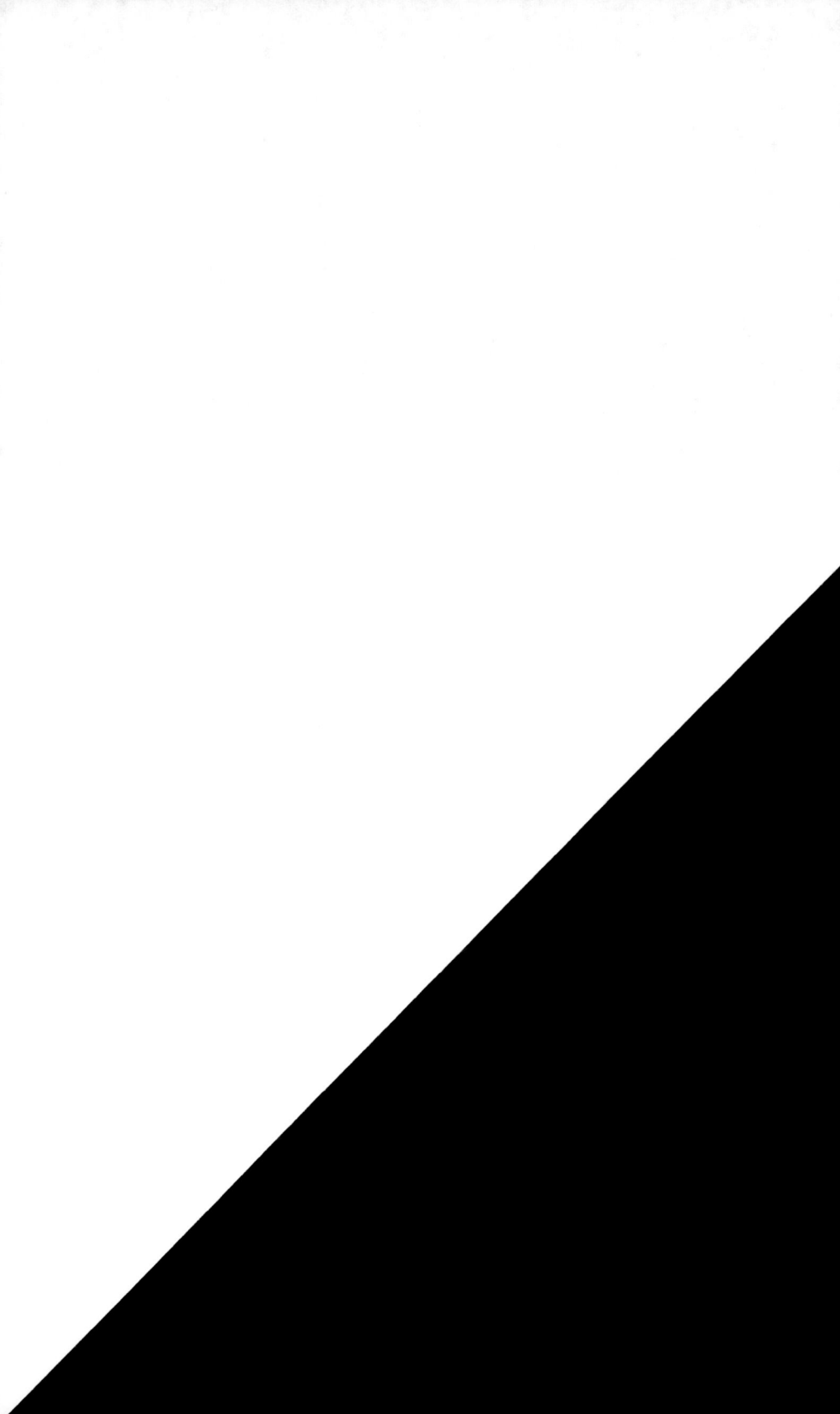